I0412289

I'm Still Here

The History, Testimony, Education, Outcomes, and Strengths of people living with HIV/AIDS

Venus Perez

© Copyright 2006 Venus Perez.
All rights reserved. No part of this publication may be reproduced, stored in a retrieval
system, or transmitted, in any form or by any means, electronic, mechanical, photocopying,
recording, or otherwise, without the written prior permission of the author.

Note for Librarians: A cataloguing record for this book is available from Library and Archives
Canada at www.collectionscanada.ca/amicus/index-e.html
ISBN 1-4251-0059-7

Printed on paper with minimum 30% recycled fibre.
Trafford's print shop runs on "green energy" from solar, wind and other environmentally-friendly power sources.

TRAFFORD
PUBLISHING™

Offices in Canada, USA, Ireland and UK

Book sales for North America and international:
Trafford Publishing, 6E–2333 Government St.,
Victoria, BC V8T 4P4 CANADA
phone 250 383 6864 (toll-free 1 888 232 4444)
fax 250 383 6804; email to orders@trafford.com
Book sales in Europe:
Trafford Publishing (UK) Limited, 9 Park End Street, 2nd Floor
Oxford, UK OX1 1HH UNITED KINGDOM
phone +44 (0)1865 722 113 (local rate 0845 230 9601)
facsimile +44 (0)1865 722 868; info.uk@trafford.com
Order online at:
trafford.com/06-1816

10 9 8 7 6 5 4 3 2

ACKNOWLEDGEMENT

I would like to thank GOD, my Lord Jesus, and the Holy Spirit for guiding my every step, and transforming my life. My husband, for his support, and kind hearted spirit, that allowed me to be me. My daughter, who is the blessing of my life. My family, and Church. My dogs, Suzie and Lola that showed me unconditional love. My best friend, PattyCake, who experienced my journey since 1987. My health care providers, who loved me and kept me alive. My present support group and my friends, (future angels I love) that allowed me to mention their names, (Randy, Lee, Becky, Baby Joey, Ed, Dennis) and past support groups throughout the years, (people I have met that are no longer with us today). And last but not least, my friend and mentor Karen Jaeger of The PLACE of comfort, who inspired and helped me blossom to the person I am today.

The thief cometh not, but for to steal, and to kill, and to destroy: I
have come that they may have life, and have it to the full.
(John 10:10) KJV

Blessings from a new generation - Madison Karen Mosey

TABLE OF CONTENTS

INTRODUCTION

The year is 2006. We have come so far yet we are not quiet there. Many lives were lost yet many still live. Many know the means of transmission, yet many, neglect to follow it. Many of us live the fast life, looking for excitement, for success. We are constantly searching for that missing part that dwells deep inside, each one of us. For many of us, we are lost, broken, unloved, discriminated, depressed and angry. We are still in denial, shunned by society as lepers were years ago.

We are individuals with HIV/AIDS. We are part of the world, and each one of us is loved by GOD, our creator, no matter who we are, or what disease we may have. We are part of this world, and this society. Our lives have meaning, and each one of us can make a difference. I would like to take you on a journey, where you can experience the history, the struggles, trials and outcomes. Our testimonies, weaknesses, strengths, and our never ending hope for tomorrow.

CHAPTER 1

SNAPSHOTS OF MODERN
HIV/AIDS

HIV (human immunodeficiency virus) is the virus that causes AIDS. This virus may be passed from one person to another when infected blood, semen, or vaginal secretions come in contact with an uninfected person's broken skin or mucous membranes*. In addition, infected pregnant women can pass HIV to their baby during pregnancy or delivery, as well as through breast-feeding. People with HIV have what is called HIV infection. Some of these people will develop AIDS as a result of their HIV infection. (-2)

1930's-1980

1930s:
Researchers believe that sometime in the 1930s a form of simian immunodeficiency virus (SIV) jumped to humans who butchered or ate chimpanzee bush meat in the Democratic Republic of Congo. The virus becomes HIV-1 the most widespread form found today. (-8)

1959:
The world's first known case of AIDS has been traced to a sample of blood plasma from a man who died in the Democratic Republic of Congo in 1959. (-8)

1960s:

HIV-2, which is restricted to West Africa, is thought to have transferred to people from sooty mangabey monkeys in Guinea-Bissau during the 1960s. (-8)

A genetic analysis of HIV in 2003 suggests that it may have first arrived in the United States in about 1968. (-8)

1970s:

During the 1970s it continues to spread undetected in the US and around the world - the pandemic has begun. (-8)

1980 –1981

December:

First case of Pneumocycstis Pneumonia (PCP) reported. (-3)

June:

First article published in MMWR on what we will later know as A.I.D.S./H.I.V. named the A Gay Cancer@. (-3)

CDC (Center for Disease Control) reports 335 cases of AIDS, with 129 deaths. (-3)

Florida:

From April 1, 1980, through June 20, 1982, 19 Haitian patients admitted to Jackson Memorial Hospital, Miami, had culture, biopsy, or autopsy evidence of opportunistic infections, and 1 other patient had biopsy- and autopsy-confirmed Kaposi's sarcoma. The infections identified included Pneumocystis carinii pneumonia (6 patients), cryptococcal meningitis or fungemia (4), toxoplasmosis of the central nervous system (CNS) (7), Candida albicans esophagitis (7) and thrush (5), esophageal or disseminated cytomegalovirus infection (3), progressive herpes simplex virus infection (1), disseminated tuberculosis (8), and chronic enteric Isospora belli infection

(2). Fourteen patients had multiple opportunistic infections. Three patients had recurring infection. The clinical course has been severe; 10 patients have died. The type of infection was initially recognized at autopsy for 6 patients. (-3)

1981:
A high prevalence of both a rare type of skin cancer - Kaposi's Sarcoma - and pneumonia are found in young gay men in New York and California, US. These are the first documented cases of AIDS. By the end of the year 121 people are known to have died from the mysterious affliction. (-8)

U.S. Centers for Disease Control and Prevention (CDC) reports first cases of rare pneumonia in young gay men, later diagnosed as AIDS-related; also issues report on highly unusual occurrence of rare skin cancer, Kaposi's Sarcoma, among young gay men. (-9)
NEW YORK TIMES publishes first news story on AIDS. (-9)

June:
On June 5, *"Pneumocystis* Pneumonia–Los Angeles," by Dr. Michael Gottlieb and colleagues of University of California at Los Angeles, appeared in *Morbidity and Mortality Weekly Report* (vol. 30, pp. 250-52), a Centers for Disease Control and Prevention (CDC) publication. This was the first article about AIDS in the medical literature. (-10)

On June 16, the first AIDS patient seen at the NIH was admitted under Dr. Thomas Waldmann's National Cancer Institute (NCI) Omnibus Metabolism Branch protocol. (-10)

July:
A Task Force on Kaposi's Sarcoma and Opportunistic Infections was established at the CDC under the direction of Dr. James Curran. (-10)

September:

On September 15, NCI sponsored a conference in Bethesda, MD, on Kaposi's Sarcoma and Opportunistic Infections. Fifty leading clinicians attended. (-10)

Fall 1981:

Simian acquired immune deficiency syndrome (simian AIDS) was identified in macaques in two of NIH's Regional Primate Centers. (-10)

Summer and Fall:

Public Health Service (PHS) agency heads discussed the new syndrome at regularly scheduled meetings. (-10)

1982

January:

On January 15–during a snowstorm that shut down the government– the second AIDS patient seen at NIH was admitted to the National Institute of Allergy and Infectious Diseases service (NIAID) and was seen by Dr. Anthony S. Fauci. (-10)

March:

First transfusion/blood related case identified. (-3)

On March 3, a conference on the new disease was held by the U.S. Public Health Service (PHS) at the CDC in Atlanta. Debate centered on whether the disease was caused by a transmissible or immune-suppressing agent(s). (-10)

NIAID intramural scientists conducted a study of adenovirus in patients with the new disease. (-10)

NCI (National Cancer Institute) established an Epidemiology Working Group on Kaposi's Sarcoma. (-10)

NCI intramural researchers conducted a field study to determine the immunological status of healthy homosexual men. (-10)

April:
Representative. Henry Waxman, (D-LA) congressman from Los Angeles, held the first congressional hearing on the new disease. The CDC estimated that tens of thousands of people would be affected by the disease. (-3) (-10)

NIAID intramural scientists studied immunoregulatory defects, herpes virus isolates, and Epstein-Barr virus and cytomegalovirus in patients with the new disease. (-10)

Mid/April:
There was a series of deaths in large cities in which stigma and isolation was attached. In these large cities this mystery disease was being called (G.R.I.D is renamed A.I.D.S) (-3)

CDC scientists name what had previously been called "Gay cancer," or more formally, GRID, (Gay Related Immuno Deficiency) AIDS (Acquired Immune Deficiency Syndrome). CDC names four risk factors: male homosexuality, intravenous drug abuse, Haitian origin and hemophilia A. (-9)

Centers for Disease Control and Prevention (CDC) scientists, in Atlanta, US, predict that the immune system disorder affecting gay men is due to an infection. They establish the term Acquired Immune Deficiency Syndrome (AIDS) and determine that aside from gay men, other groups at risk are injecting drug users, people of Haitian origin and haemophiliacs. (-8)

By 1982 AIDS had been detected on five continents. (-8)

It is revealed that a wasting disorder known in Africa as "slim disease" is a form of AIDS. (-8)

Center for Disease Control says sexual contact or infected blood could transmit AIDS. (-9)

First U.S. Congressional hearings held on HIV/AIDS. (-9)

Gay Men's Health Crisis, (GMHC) established in New York City. (-9)

June:
NIH Clinical Center (CC) protocol approved to study etiology of immunoregulatory defects in the new disease as a collaborative effort among CC departments, NIAID, NCI, National Institute of Neurological Diseases and Communicative Disorders and Stroke (NINCDS), National Institute of Dental Research (NIDR), National Eye Institute (NEI), and the Food and Drug Administration (FDA). (-10)

An NIH Working Group to study the new disease was established with representatives from each institute and liaisons from the CDC and FDA. (-10)

NINCDS investigators provided clinical appraisal of neurological symptoms in CC protocols. (-10)

NINCDS collaborated on studies of simian AIDS. (-10)

The National Library of Medicine (NLM) began to compile a bibliography on manifestations of the new disease. (-10)

On June 30, persuasive evidence that the disease was caused by an infectious agent was presented at a meeting held at the New York Department of Health: cases had been reported in intravenous drug users, homosexuals, hemophiliacs, and Haitians. (-10)

July 15:
The CDC reported 413 cases of the new disease in the United States with 155 deaths. (-10)

July 27:
At a meeting in Washington, DC, attended by federal officials, university researchers, community activists, and others, the name "acquired immune deficiency syndrome," or AIDS, was selected for the new disease. (-10)

August:
NCI issued a Request for Applications (RFA) for research projects related to AIDS. Six grants for this RFA were awarded by NCI and NIAID in May 1983. (-10)

September:
The CDC reported 593 cases of AIDS in the United States with 243 deaths. (-10)

The CDC defined a case of AIDS as a disease, at least moderately predictive of a defect in cell-mediated immunity, occurring in a person with no known cause for diminished resistance to that disease. (-10)

November:
The CDC published formal recommendations for the protection of laboratory and clinical personnel having contact with AIDS patients and clinical specimens. The recommendations were based on those for hepatitis B. (-10)

The National Heart, Lung, and Blood Institute (NHLBI) signed an intra-agency agreement with CDC to evaluate immunological alterations following transfusion with blood or blood products in people with hemophilia, sickle-cell disease, and thalassemia. (-10)

December:
Children that were given blood transfusions were now found with this disease. The virus has now entered the blood supply. (CDC reports 1,201 cases of A.I.D.S., with 466 deaths. (-3)

First hemophilia related case identified. (-3)

The CDC reported a case of AIDS caused by blood transfusion in a previously healthy infant (First documented case). (-3) (-10)

Later that month the first reports appeared that the disease was occurring in Haitians, as well as hemophiliacs. (-7)

By the beginning of July a total of 452 cases, from 23 states, had been reported to the CDC. (-5)

NIH's intramural study of the natural history of the immunodeficiency and consequent opportunistic infections had enrolled 25 patients with AIDS (-10)

1983

January:
First reported case of A.I.D.S in a female partner of a male with A.I.D.S. (-3)

The CDC met with blood banking organizations in Atlanta to discuss proposals to screen out individuals at high risk for AIDS from the blood donor pool. Self-identification through questionnaires or interviews was proposed. (-10)

Mid:
Safer sex guidelines are proposed. (-3)

March:
NHLBI convened a meeting of scientific experts to formulate research recommendations for studies on AIDS and blood transfusion. (-10)
Epidemiological evidence showed that AIDS primarily affected gay men in San Francisco and New York City. In New Jersey, AIDS patients were primarily intravenous drug users and Haitians, and 68 percent of cases were in African Americans or Latinos. (-10)

The CDC published guidelines adopted by the PHS requesting members of groups having increased risk for AIDS to refrain from donating blood. (-10)

Spring:
At the invitation of the Haitian Ministry of Health, Dr. Richard Krause, NIAID director, led a small delegation of NIAID and CDC scientists to Haiti to study the AIDS epidemic there and assist their clinicians. (-10)

NIAID hosted a major meeting of experts in Bethesda, Maryland, to discuss possible etiologies of AIDS. Dr. Albert Sabin summarized the meeting, urging researchers to "cast a wide net." (-10)

May:
Dr. Luc Montagnier and his collaborators at the Pasteur Institute reported in *Science* isolating a new retrovirus, LAV, associated with AIDS; they did not claim LAV caused AIDS. (-10)

June:
The CDC reported 1,641 cases of AIDS in the United States with 644 deaths. (-10)

The NIH Clinical Center issued precautions for health care workers caring for AIDS patients. (-10)

July:
NIAID awarded contracts to the New York Blood Center and the Memorial Sloan Kettering Cancer Center to collect specimens from AIDS patients to look for the etiologic agent. (-10)

Summer:
The U.S. Department of Health and Human Services (DHHS) issued several statements seeking to calm public fears that AIDS could be contracted casually. (-10)

August:
NIAID began publishing an informal newsletter, the *AIDS Memorandum*, through which scientists could share unpublished research findings. This publication lasted for two years until AIDS articles were given expedited publication by mainstream journals. (-10)

September:
NIDR issued recommendations to practicing dentists about precautions they should take in managing their patients with AIDS. (-10)

The CDC reported 2,259 cases of AIDS in the United States with 917 deaths. (-10)

On September 12-13, the NIH Workshop on the Epidemiology of AIDS was held at the Holiday Inn Crowne Plaza in Rockville, Maryland. (-10)

NIAID and NCI launched the Multicenter AIDS Cohort Study (MACS) and the San Francisco Men's Health Study (SFMHS) to develop large, comprehensive, longitudinal studies of populations that seemed to be at risk of AIDS. Soon thereafter, NIAID assumed complete responsibility for the program. (-10)

October:
Projet SIDA, a multidisciplinary study based in Kinshasa, Zaire, was initiated jointly by NIAID, CDC, the Belgian Institute of Tropical Medicine, and the Zairean Ministry of Health. (-10)

December:
CDC reports 3,153 cases of A.I.D.S., with 1,512 deaths. (-3)

Late:
AIDS budget to $4.3 million. (-3)

AIDS epidemics are developing in Europe: one in gay men who have visited the US, another in people with links to central Africa. (-8)

Investigations begin into the occurrence of AIDS in Rwanda, Zaire and other African nations. (-8)

The Orphan Drug Act is signed into U.S. law, providing incentives to drug companies to develop therapies for rare diseases. (-9)

U.S. CDC adds female sexual partners of men with AIDS as fifth risk group. (-9)

People living with AIDS (PWAs) issue The Denver Principles. (-9)

1984

January:
The CDC reported 3,000 cases of AIDS in the United Sates with 1,283 deaths. (-10)

NHLBI convened an Ad Hoc Working Group on AIDS and Blood Transfusions. (-10)

April:
HTLV-III discovered as cause for A.I.D.S., modes of transmission identified. (-3)

On April 23, DHHS held a press conference where HHS Secretary Margaret Heckler announced that Dr. Robert Gallo of NCI had found the cause of AIDS, the retrovirus HTLV-III. She also announced the development of a diagnostic blood test to identify HTLV-III and expressed hope that a vaccine against AIDS could be produced within two years. (-10)

May:

Four papers from Dr. Gallo's laboratory demonstrating that the HTLV-III retrovirus was the cause of AIDS were published in *Science*. (-10)

NHLBI awarded a contract to establish a volunteer blood donor serum repository for HTLV-III donor/recipient studies. (-10)

NHLBI, CDC, and FDA cosponsored an AIDS ethics conference. (-10)

NIDR intramural investigators showed that the AIDS virus can infect not only T4 lymphocytes but also macrophages. (-10)

Mid:

CDC redefines case definition for A.I.D.S to in clued opportunistic infections. (-3)

June

Drs. Robert Gallo and Luc Montagnier held a joint press conference to announce that Gallo's HTLV-III virus and Montagnier's LAV were almost certainly identical. (-10)

The CDC reported 4,918 cases of AIDS in the United States with 2,221 deaths. (-10)

The CDC reported 4,918 cases of AIDS in the United States with 2,221 deaths. (-10)

Summer:

Intensive study of the AIDS retrovirus was launched, resulting in findings such as: the CD4 molecule on T4 helper lymphocytes was identified as one receptor by which the AIDS virus entered cells. Genetic sequences of HTLV-III and LAV were determined. (-10)

Sept:

A meeting between NCI investigators and Burroughs Welcome pharmaceutical company was held to discuss plans to test potential drugs as retrovirus inhibitors. The outcome of this meeting was research and development of AZT, the first anti-retroviral drug approved to treat AIDS. (-10)

AZT first considered for use. (-3)

November:

On November 2, Dr. Anthony S. Fauci was named NIAID director. (-10)

Pasteur Institute investigators published the genetic sequence of LAV. (-10)

The CDC reported 6,993 cases of AIDS in the United States with 3,342 deaths. (-10)

Fall:

NIAID held a conference at its Rocky Mountain Laboratories in Hamilton, Montana, on potential animal models for retrovirus infections and their relationship to AIDS. (-10)

Dec:

Ryan White, 13, diagnosed with A.I.D.S. and barred from school the following year. (-3)

CDC reports 6,360 cases of A.I.D.S., with 3,518 deaths.   (-3)

Using recently developed techniques, the retrovirus responsible for AIDS is independently discovered by Luc Montagnier of the Pasteur Institute in Paris, France, and Robert Gallo of the National Cancer Institute in Washington DC, US. It is later named the human immunodeficiency virus (HIV). (-8)

Cases of AIDS passed on through heterosexual intercourse begin to appear. (-8)

CDC states that abstention from intravenous drug use and reduction of needle-sharing "should also be effective in preventing transmission of the virus." (-9)

1985

January:
On January 17, NCI scientists and their collaborators published the genome of HTLV-III in *Nature*. (-10)

March:
Blood banks begin testing donated blood after FDA approves antibody test. (-3)
1st HTLV-III antibody test released. (-3)
On March 7, the first AIDS antibody test, an ELISA-type test, was released. (-10)

April:
On April 15-17, the first International AIDS Conference was held in Atlanta, sponsored by NIH, CDC, and FDA; the Alcohol, Drug Abuse, and Mental Health Administration; the Health Resources and Services Administration; and the World Health Organization (WHO). An international network of Collaborating Centers on AIDS was formed. (-10)

May:
A.R.C. (medical term denoting "A.I.D.S. Related Complex") is first used, and then abandoned. (-3)

The CDC reported 10,000 cases of AIDS in the United States with 4,942 deaths. (-10)

First Anonymous Test Sites opened. (-3)

Mid:

$106.5 million spent in A.I.D.S research. (-3)

June:

1st International A.I.D.S. Conference held in Atlanta, GA. (-3)
The CDC revised the case definition of AIDS to include additional specific disease conditions and to exclude people as AIDS cases if they had a negative result on testing for serum antibody to HTLV-III/LAV. (-10)

July:

Rock Hudson discloses he has A.I.D.S and dies in October. (-3)

United Press International reported that actor Rock Hudson had AIDS. (-10)

Aug:

AIDS becomes the #1 health problem. (-3)

91% of all insurance companies deny coverage to H.I.V infected patients. (-3)

14 year- old Ryan White diagnosed and barred from school. (-3)

Late:

Vice-President Bush says A.I.D.S is an epidemic. (-3)

CDC reports 12,026 cases of A.I.D.S., with 6,997 deaths. (-3)

Cumulatively, CDC reports 23,174 cases of A.I.D.S., with 12,652 deaths. (-3)

The first International AIDS conference is held in Atlanta, US. (-8)

Following the previous year's discovery of the HIV virus, the first HIV test is licensed by the US Food and Drug Administration (FDA). (-8)

US blood banks are screened for the virus. (-8)

First International AIDS Conference held in Atlanta. Hosted by U.S. Department of Health and Human Services (DHHS) and the World Health Organization (WHO). (-9)

FDA approved first enzyme linked immunosorbant assay (ELISA) test kit to screen for antibodies to HIV. (-9)

Project Inform founded to advocate for faster government approval of HIV drugs. (-9)

The U.S. Public Health Service issues first recommendations for preventing transmission of HIV from mother to child. (-9)

American foundation for AIDS Research (amfAR) is founded by Co-Chairs Mathilde Krim and Michael S. Gottlieb, and National Chair Elizabeth Taylor. (-9)

Pentagon announces that it will begin testing all new recruits for HIV infection and will reject those who are positive. (-9)

Sept:
Indiana teen Ryan White, a hemophiliac suffering from AIDS, was refused entry to school. (-10)

The U.S. military services began testing for the AIDS virus among its personnel. (-10)

October:
Rock Hudson died on October 2. He was the first major public figure to die of AIDS. Public fear about AIDS increased dramatically. (-10)

December:
Publication of a finding that the AIDS virus is present in saliva increased public fears about AIDS. (-10)

1986

January:
The CDC reported 16,458 cases of AIDS in the United Sates with 8,361 deaths. (-10)

February:
NIAID established a Division of AIDS. (-10)

April:
Every 14 hours a San Franciscan dies. (-3)

May:
HTLV-III renamed H.I.V. (-3)

Surgeon General Koop releases report calling for A.I.D.S education for children and widespread use of condoms. (-3)

The name of the AIDS virus was changed to human immunodeficiency virus (HIV) at the suggestion of a multinational committee of scientists.

June:
At a PHS-sponsored conference at the Coolfont Conference Center in West Virginia, a prediction was made that in 2001, some 270,000 people in the United States would have been diagnosed with AIDS and that 179,000 would have died. (-10)

NIAID established AIDS Treatment Evaluation Units (ATEUs), which later became AIDS Clinical Trials Units (ACTUs). (-10)

July:
NHLBI cosponsored with FDA and the NIH Office on Medical Applications of Research a conference on the "Impact of HTLV-III Antibody Testing on the Public Health." (-10)

Sept:

Large scale information and dissemination on treatments by groups such as Project inform. (-3)

October:

The CDC reported that although the incidence of AIDS was rising for all racial/ethnic groups and in all geographic regions of the country, the cumulative incidence of AIDS among blacks and Hispanics was more than three times the rate for whites. (-10)

Surgeon General C. Everett Koop released his "Report on Acquired Immune Deficiency." (-10)

Dec:

The CDC reported 28,098 cases of AIDS in the United States with 15,757 deaths. (-10)

Ronald Reagan mentions AIDS on February 6, 1986, vowing in a letter to Congress to make AIDS a priority. (-9)

Institute of Medicine report calls for a national education campaign and creation of National Commission on AIDS. (-9)

U.S. Surgeon General Koop issues "Surgeon General's Report on AIDS", calling for education and condom use. (-9)

National Academy of Science issues report critical of the U.S. response to "national health crisis;" calls for a $2 billion investment. (-9)

Robert Wood Johnson Foundation creates "AIDS Health Services Program", providing funding to hard hit U.S. cities; program is precursor to Ryan White CARE Act. (-9)

1987

Jan:

Statistics show that 50% of all HIV cases will progress to A.I.D.S. (-3)

WHO (World Health Organization) launches Global Program for A.I.D.S. (-3) (-10)

Feb:

Plan for H.I.V quarantine proposed in California. (-3)

WHO (World Health Organization) launches Global Program for A.I.D.S. (-3) (-10)

Mar:

FDA approves AZT- the first antiretroviral drug, used as a cancer drug in the 1950's produced an unexpected response to the HIV virus (AZT approved for use.) (-3) (-10)

AZT (zidovudine), the first antiretroviral drug, becomes available to treat HIV sufferers after a successful clinical trial. The drug works by blocking the action of HIV's enzyme reverse transcriptase, stopping the virus from replicating in cells. AZT slows down the course of AIDS, delaying death. (-8)

 By 1987, 16,908 people have died from AIDS in the US. In total 71,751 cases of AIDS had been reported to the World Health Organization (WHO), 47,022 in the US. (-8)

Estimating that as many as 5 to 10 million people could be infected with HIV worldwide, the WHO launches its Global Programme on AIDS. (-8)

FDA approved AZT- the first drug approved for the treatment of AIDS. (-9)

FDA pulbishes regulations which require screeing all bllod and plasma collected in the U.S. for HIV antibodies. (-9)

FDA revised its strategy for the regulation of condoms by strenghening its inspection of condom manufacturers and repackers, strengthening its sampling and testing of domestic and imported condoms in commerical distribution, and providing guidance on labeling of condoms for the prevention of AIDS. (-9)

The AIDS Drug Assistance Program (ADAP) is initiated to ensure the availability of medications to un- or under-insured PWA's (People with AIDS). (-9)

Global Programe on AIDS launched by the World Health Organization. (-9)

President Reagan establishes the Presidential Commission on HIV (Watkins commission). (-9)

President Ronald Reagan and French Prime Minister Jacques Chirac announced a joint agreement settling the dispute arising from the discovery of the AIDS virus, the first international agreement relating to a biomedical research issue to be announced by heads of state. (-10)

U.S adds HIV as a "dangerous contagious disease" to its immigration exclusion list; mandates testing of all applicants. (-9)

U.S CDC holds its first National Conference on HIV and communities of color. (-9)

U.S. FDA creates new class of experimental drugs, Treatment Investigational New Drugs (INDs), which accelerates drug approval by two to three years. (-9)

U. S. Congress approves $30 million in emergency funding to states for AZT.

U.S. Congress adopts Helms Amendment banning use of feder funds for AIDS education materials that "promote or encourage, directly or indirectly, homosexual activities," often referred to as the "no promo homo" policy. (-9)

U.S CDC launches first AIDS-related public service announcements, "America Responds to AIDS". (-9)

April:
FDA approved the first Western blot blood test–a more specific HIV diagnostic test. (-10)

May:
The CDC reported that between 1981 and 1987, nine health care workers caring for AIDS patients and having no other risk factors had been infected with HIV. (-10)

June:
NHLBI awarded a contract to maintain a colony of 50 chimpanzees for studies of post-transfusion HIV infection and AIDS. (-10)

August:
The CDC reported 40,051 cases of AIDS in the United States with 23,165 deaths. (-10)

On August 18, Dr. H. Clifford Lane and his NIAID colleagues began the first U.S. clinical trial at NIH to test an experimental HIV vaccine in humans. (-10)

NIAID established the AIDS Vaccine Evaluation Group (AVEG), a network of clinical sites to conduct trials of experimental HIV vaccines. (-10)

Fall:
The NIH Office of the Director launched its Targeted Antiviral Program to encourage intramural analysis of the three-dimensional

structure of HIV and to determine the shape of protein-bound drugs. (-10)

October:
Cleve Jones made the first panel for the AIDS Memorial Quilt in memory of his friend Marvin Feldman. (-10)
NIAID established 17 Clinical Study Groups (CSGs) to extend to a wider geographical area access to clinical trials of promising AIDS therapies. (-10)

December:
The CDC released the results of a study on the prevalence of HIV infection in the United States, indicating a shifting emphasis toward defining AIDS as "infection with HIV" rather than by defining particular "indicator diseases" that characterized late-stage AIDS. (-10)

1988

January:
The CDC updated the International Classification of Diseases codes for HIV infection for use with U.S. morbidity and mortality data. (-10)
The CDC published guidelines developed for educational efforts to combat AIDS. (-10)

February:
On February 12, trimetrexate was the first AIDS drug granted pre-approval distribution status under new FDA regulations. The drug was used to treat *Pneumocystis carinii* pneumonia in AIDS patients who could not tolerate standard treatments. (-10)

March:
A total of 136 countries or territories reported a total of 84,256 cases of AIDS to the WHO Global Programme on AIDS. (-10)

April:

The NIH reported that between 1981 and 1988, two workers in laboratories producing large quantities of HIV had been infected with HIV, and it issued biosafety recommendations for laboratories. (-10) NIAID established an AIDS reagent repository to catalogue and expedite the availability of experimental materials used in AIDS research. (-10)

June:

The CDC reported that a new AIDS case was reported every 14 minutes. (-10)

The brochure "Understanding AIDS," prepared by Surgeon General C. Everett Koop in collaboration with the CDC, was mailed to every household in the United States. (-10)

NIAID and NICHD established an epidemiologic study of HIV transmission during pregnancy and birth, the Women and Infants Transmission Study (WITS). (-10)

August:

The CDC reported 72,024 cases of AIDS in the United States and estimated that 1 to 1.5 million Americans were infected with HIV. (-10)

NIAID's AIDS Vaccine Evaluation Units initiated their first study of an experimental AIDS vaccine. (-10)

September:

The World Health Organization reported that 111,000 cases of AIDS had been documented worldwide. Authorities at WHO placed the actual number of cases, including those unreported, at 250,000. (-10)

NIDR investigators reported that saliva inhibits transmission of HIV. (-10)

October:

AIDS protestors, demanding a quicker approval process for drug treatments, shut down the FDA. (-10)

On October 13, NIAID established three programs: the Centers for AIDS Research (CFARS) to improve the diagnosis, treatment, and prevention of AIDS; the Pediatric AIDS Clinical Trials Units (Pediatric ACTUs), a network of clinical sites to test experimental HIV drugs in children; and the Programs for Excellence in Basic Research (PEBRA), to develop novel strategies to determine how HIV causes disease. (-10)

November:

NIAID established the International Collaborations in AIDS Research (ICAR) program to encourage studies of AIDS in Africa, Mexico, and Brazil. (-10)

NIAID established the Clinical Programs for Clinical Research on AIDS (CPCRA) to involve community physicians in AIDS research. (-10)

A CDC study revealed that 3 of every 1,000 college students are infected with HIV. (-10)

The NIH Office of AIDS Research (OAR) was established. (-10)

On November 21, FDA licensed Intron A and Roferon A (human alpha interferon injection) for the treatment of Kaposi's sarcoma. (-10)

On November 28, FDA authorized pre-approval distribution of ganciclovir under a treatment IND protocol for the treatment of cytomegalovirus retinitis in AIDS patients. (-10)

December:

NIAID funds a natural history study, HATS, in male and female heterosexuals at high risk of AIDS who are not IV drug users. The study is modeled on the MACS. (-10)

On December 1, WHO's (World Health Organization) Global Programme on AIDS instituted the first World AIDS Day as an annual event on December 1. (-8) (-10)

On December 22, Dr. Samuel Broder was named NCI director. (-10)

FDA implemented new regulations designed to make promising therapies available sooner. Subpart E of the IND regulations established procedures designed to expedite development, evaluation, and marketing of new therapies intended to treat patients with life-threatening and severely-debilitating diseases. (-9)

The U.S. Healthe Omnibus Programs Extension (HOPE) Act of 1988 authorizes the use of federal funds for AIDS prevention, education, and testing. (-9)

U. S FDA allows the importation of unapproved drugs for persons with life-threatening illnesses, including HIV/AIDS. (-9)

U.S Surgeon General and CDC mail brochure, "Understanding AIDS" to all U.S. households; first and only national mailing of its kind. (-9)

U.S National Institutes of Health (NIH) establishes Office of AIDS Research (OAR) and AIDS Clinical Trials Group (ACTG). (-9)

1989

U. S Congress creates the National commission on AIDS. (-9)

February 3:
FDA authorized pre-approval distribution of aerosolized pentamidine under a treatment IIND protocol for the prevention of Pneumocystis carinii pneumonia. (-12)

June 15:
FDA approved NebPent (aerosolized pentamidine) for the prevention of Pneumocystis Carinii pneumonia. (-12)

June 23:
FDA approved Cytoven (ganciclovir) infusion for use in the treatment of cytomegalovirus Retinal infections in persons with AIDS. (-12)

June 27:
FDA authorized pre-approval distribution of erythropoietin (EPO) under a treatment IND protocol for the treatment of zidovudine (AZT) related anemia in HIV positive patients. (-12)

September 28:
FDA approved Retrovir (zidovudine, AZT) in syrup formulation. (-12)

FDA authorized pre-approval distribution of dideoxyinosine (ddI) under a treatment IND protocol for the treatment of patients with AIDS or AIDS Related Complex who are intolerant to zidovudine (AZT). (-12)

FDA licensed the first diagnostic kit to detect the presence of HIV-1 by directly detecting the proteins, or antigens, of the virus. (-12)

FDA participated in the establishment of an AIDS Clinical Trial Information Service (ACTIS), a computerized listing of information on AIDS-related clinical trials available via toll free telephone service. (-12)

October 26:
FDA authorized pre-approval distribution of Retrovir (zidovudine, AZT) under a treatment IND protocol for the treatment of pediatric patients with HIV disease. (-12)

1990

January 29:
FDA approved Diflucan (fluconazole) tablets to treat two serious AIDS-related fungal infections (Cryptococcal meningitis and candidiasis). (-12)

February 2:
FDA approved Retrovir (zidovudine, AZT) in an intravenous dosage form. (-12)

Expanded labeling for Retrovir (zidovudine, AZT) was approved, including dosage (January 1990), for use in early HIV disease (March 1990), and for use with children (May 1990). (-12)

December 12:
FDA published a final rule defining acceptable quality levels for medical gloves and establishing the sampling plans and test methods that FDA will use to determine whether gloves are adulterated. (-12)

December 31:
FDA approved Epogen (erythropoietin, EPO) for the treatment of zidovudine-related anemia. (-12)

FDA granted a license for the Recombigen HIV-1 EIA HIV antibody detection kit, designed for high volume screening sites. (-12)

FDA approved Novopath HIV-1 Immunoblot test for the detection of antibodies to individual proteins of HIV-1. This test is nearly 5 times faster than comparable tests using the same technology. (-12)

At the beginning of the year, it was reported that a large number of children in Romanian hospitals and orphanages had become infected with HIV as a result of multiple blood transfusions and the reuse of needles. Jonathan Mann, the head of WHO's Global programme on

AIDS, noted that 'Eastern Europe is the new frontier for the AIDS epidemic'.(-11)

"Jonathan's persistence and passion helped wake up the world."(-15)

"Had it not been for Jonathan's unique contributions, the world's approach to AIDS might very well have gone towards mandatory testing and quarantine."(-16)

6th International AIDS Conference ("AIDS in the Nineties: From Science to Policy"),

San Francisco, CA. To protest U.S. immigration policy, domestic and international non-Governmental groups boycott the conference. (-9)

Ryan White dies at the age of 18. The Ryan White Comprehensive AIDS Resources Emergency (CARE) Act of 1990 is enacted by the U.S. Congress. The Act Provides Federal funds for community-based care and treatment services. Critics contend the Act is under-funded. (-9)

Americans with Disabilities Act of 1990 by the U.S. congress, pro-hibiting discrimination again individuals with disabilities, including people living with HIV/AIDS. (-9)

American AIDS deaths pass the 10,000. (-9)

1991

The red ribbon becomes an international symbol of AIDS aware-ness. (-8)

CDC recommends restrictions on the practice of HIV-positive health care workers and Congress enacts law requiring states to take simi-lar action. (-9)

Housing Opportunities for People with AIDS (HOPWA) Act of 1991 enacted, providing grants to U.S. states and local communities. (-9)

ICASO (International council of AIDS Service Organizations) forms. (-9)

New York City Board of Education approves an HIV/AIDS initiative, which includes condom availability in high schools. (-9)

1992

In the US, AIDS becomes the leading cause of death for 24 to 44 year old men. (-8)

The first combination drug therapies for HIV are introduced, when the US FDA approves the use of the ddC, which also blocks reverse transcriptase, alongside AZT. HIV drug cocktails are more effective and the multi-pronged attacks slow down the development of drug resistance. (-8)

8th Internation AIDS Conferenc ("A World United Against AIDS"), Amsterdam, would have taken place in Boston, but was moved due to U.S immigration ban. (-9)

AIDS becomes number one cause of death for U.S men ages 25 to 44. (-9)

A federal court strikes down " offensiveness" restrictions on AIDS education materials proposed by Senator Jesse Helms. (-9)

1993

President Clinton establishes White House Office of National AIDS Policy (ONAP). (-9)

Women's Interagency HIV Study (WIHS) and HIV Epidemiology Study (HERS) begin; both major U.S. Federally-funded research studies on women and HIV/AIDS. (-9)

U.S. Congress enacts the NIH Revitalization Act, giving the OAR primary oversight of all NIH AIDS research; requires NIH and other research agencies to expand involvement of women and minorities in all research. (-9)

First annual "AIDSWatch"- hundreds of community members from acrouss the U.S.

Converge in Washington, DC to lobby Congress for increased AIDS funding. (-9)

President Clinton signs HIV immigration exclusion policy into law. (-9) The CDC, NIH, and FDA declare in a joint statement that condoms are "highly Effective" for prevention of HIV infection. (-9)

1994

Using AZT to reduce the transmission of HIV from pregnant women to unborn fetuses is recommended in the US. A study shows it cuts the rate of maternal transmission to 8% - in women taking a placebo the rate was 25%. (-8)

Over 12 after the discovery of AIDS, the US government launches its first national media campaign explicitly promoting condoms. (-8)

U.S. FDA approves an oral HIV test, the first non-blood based anti-body test for HIV, (-9)

AIDS becomes leading cause of death for all Americans ages 25 to 44; remains so through 1995. (-9)

1995

First protease inhibitor drug, saquinavir, approved in record time by the U.S. FDA, highly active antiretroviral therapy (HAART) becomes available to treat. (-8) (-9)

HIV. These drugs result in defective HIV forming, which cannot infect new cells. This new more powerful drug heralds the start of Highly Active Antiretroviral Therapy (HAART) - a combination therapy regimen using a "cocktail" of drugs. (-8)

One million cases of AIDS have been reported to the WHO, 19.5 million people have been infected with HIV since the epidemic began. (-8)

First White House Conference on HIV/AIDS. (-9)

First National HIV Testing Day created by the National Association of People with AIDS. (-9)

1996

The International AIDS Vaccine Initiative (IAVI) - a non-profit organisation based in New York City - is set up to speed the search for an HIV vaccine. (-8)

90% of all people infected with HIV now live in the developing world. (-8)

Ronald Reagan mentions AIDS on Feb. 6, 1986, vowing in a letter to Congress make AIDS a priority. (-9)

Joint United Nations Programme on HIV/AIDS (UNAIDS) begins operations. (-9)

U.S. FDA approves first non-nucleoside reverse transcriptase inhibitor (NNRTI), nevirapine. (-9)

HIV no longer leading cause of death for all Americans ages 35-44; remains leading cause of death for African Americans in this age group. Annual US death rates from AIDS dramatically fall for the first time, due to the introduction of HAART. (-8)

UN announces that 40 million children could have lost one or both parents to AIDS by 2010. (-8)

WHO estimates that 30.6 million peoplel are living with HIV/AIDS worldwide, more than the population of Australia. (-9)

The Levine Committee, a blue ribbon advisory panel, calls for overhaul of NIH AIDS research, including stronger role for OAR and increased support for caccine-related and investigator-initiated reseach. (-9)

Brazil begins national ARV distribution, first developing county to do so. (-9)

The number of new AIDS cases diagnosed in the U.S. declines for first time in history of epidemic, though experience varies by sex, race, and ethnicity. (-9)

Internation AIDS Vaccine Initiative (IAVI), an AGO, forms to speed the search for an effective HIV vaccine. (-9)

1997

AIDS-related deaths in the U.S. decline by more than 40 percent compared to the prior year, largely due to HAART. (-9)

President Clinton announces goal of finding an effective vaccine in 10 years and the creation of Dale and Betty Bumpers Vaccine Research Center. (-9)

U.S. Congress enacts FDA Modernization Act of 1997, codifying accelerated approval process, and allowing dissemination of information about off-label uses of drugs. (-9)

Annual US death rates from AIDS dramatically fall for the first time, due to the introduction of HAART. (-8)

UN announces that 40 million children could have lost one or both parents to AIDS by 2010. (-8)

WHO estimates that 30.6 million peoplel are living with HIV/AIDS worldwide, more than the population of Australia. (-9)

1998

The first full-scale trial of a vaccine against HIV begins in the US. (-8)

Two teams of researchers begin developing vaccines targeted against the strains of HIV prevalent in sub-Saharan Africa. (-8)

An HIV strain resistant to all protease inhibitor drugs currently on the market turns up in San Francisco. Unusual side effects, such as the growth of fatty pads and heart problems, are occurring in some users of protease inhibitors. (-8)

AIDS is now New York City's leading cause of death for women ages 25 to 44. (-9)

U.S. Department of Health and Human Services Secretary Shalala determines that needle exchange programs are effective and do not encourage the use of illegal drugs, but Clinton Administration does not lift the ban on use of federal funds for such purposes. (-9)

The U.S. Supreme Court in Bragdon v. Abbott rules that the Americans with Disabilities Act covers those in earlier stages of HIV disease, not just AIDS. (-9)

Ricky Ray Hemophila Relief Fund Act of 1998 enacted by U.S. Congress, authorizing payments to hemophiliacs infected through unscreened blood-clotting agents between 1982 and 1987. (-9)

First large scale human trials (Phase III) for an HIV vaccine begin. (-9)

Minority AIDS AIDS Initiative created in U.S., after African American leaders declare a "state of emergency" and Congressional Black

Caucus (CBC) calls on the Department of Health and Human Services to do the same. (-9)

1999

Edward Hooper releases his book, *The River*, which accuses doctors who tested a polio vaccine in 1950s Africa of unintentionally starting the AIDS epidemic. The idea is rejected in 2001 by a wide group of researchers. (-8)

33 million people are infected with HIV, and 14 million have died of AIDS worldwide. (-8)

AIDS becomes the fourth biggest killer worldwide. (-8)

First human vaccine trial in a developing country begins in Thailand. (-9)

President Clinton announces "Leadership and Investment in Fighting an Epidemic" (LIFE) Initiative to address the global epidemic; leads to increased funding. (-9)

2000

New York State passes legislation decriminalizing sale and possession of syringes without prescription. (-9)

U.S. Department of Health and Human Services approves first state 1115 Medicaid expansion waivers for low-income people with HIV. (-9)

President Clinton creates first ever Presidential Envoy for AIDS Cooperation. (-9)

President Clinton announces Millennium Vaccine Initiative, creating incentives for development and distribution of vaccines against HIV, TB and malaria. (-9)

Global AIDS and Tuberculosis Relief Act of 2000 enacted by U.S. Congress, authorizing up to $600 million for U.S. global efforts. (-9)

UNAIDS, WHO and other global health groups announce joint initiative with five major pharmaceutical manufacturers to negotiate reduced prices for AIDS drugs in developing countries. (-9)

G8 Leaders acknowledge need for additional HIV/AIDS resources during Okinawa Meeting. (-9)

U.S. CDC forms Global AIDS Program (GAP). (-9)

Millennium Development Goals, announced as part of Millennium Declaration, include reversing the spread of HIV/AIDS, malaria and TB as one of 8 key goals. (-9)

President Clinton issues Executive Order to assist developing countries in importing and producing generic forms of HIV treatments. (-9)

U.S. and UN Security Councils declare HIV/AIDS a security threat. (-9)

13th International AIDS Conference ("Breaking the Silence"), Durban, South Africa; first to be held in a developing nation, heightens awareness of the global pandemic. (-9)

2001

An Indian company starts to sell discounted copies of expensive patented AIDS drugs to a medical charity in Africa. The move forces some pharmaceutical companies to slash prices. (-8)

The 189 member nations of the U.N. General Assembly adopt by consensus a global blueprint for action on HIV/AIDS and Secretary General Kofi Annan calls for the creation of a $7 to $10 billion global fund to combat AIDS in the developing world. (-9)

A new study shows that 14% of individuals newly infected with HIV in the U.S. already exhibit resistance to at least one antiviral drug. (-9)

Generic drug manufacturers offer to produce discounted, generic forms of HIV/AIDS drugs; several major pharmaceutical manufacturers agree to offer further reduced drugs prices in developing countries. (-9)

The World Trade Organization, announces "DOHA Agreement", to allow developing countries to buy or manufacture generic medications to meet public health crises, such as HIV/AIDS. (-9)

U.S. Secretary of State, Colin Powell, reaffirms U.S. statement that HIV/AIDS is a national security threat. (-9)

United Nations General Assembly convenes first ever special session on AIDS, "UNGASS" UN Secretary-General Kofi Annan calls for a global fund, a "war chest", to fight AIDS, during African Summit on HIV/AIDS in Abuja, Nigeria. (-9)

2002

February:

Franklin Graham-The son of legendary evangelist Billy Graham, Rev. Franklin Graham heads Samaritan's Purse, a nondenominational evangelical Christian charity dedicated to providing spiritual and material aid to victims of war, poverty, natural disasters, disease and famine. As he realized the devastation HIV/AIDS was causing around the world, Graham, in a meeting with evangelicals -- and with Bush administration officials in the audience –called on them to put a Christian stamp on the issue and make AIDS their new cause. Here, Graham talks about the need to provide biblically-based AIDS education and prevention efforts, and recounts how he advised former Sen. Jesse Helms (R.-N.C.) to embrace people living with HIV/AIDS. (-6)

The Bush Administration removes Condom Fact Sheets from the "Programs that Work" section of the HHS Website. After protests, revised Condom Fact Sheets are later reposted to the website. (-9)

The Bush Administration begins promoting abstinence-only HIV prevention programs and targets programs that do otherwise for audits by the Office of the Inspector General of the Department of Health and Human Services. (-9)

UNAIDS Reports that women comprise about half of all adults living with HIV/AIDS worldwide. (-9)

HIV is leading cause of death worldwide, among those aged 15-59. (-9)

The Global Fund to Fight AIDS, Tuberculosis, and Malaria begins operations; approves first round of grants later this year. (-9)

2003

Five million people are newly infected with AIDS during 2003, the greatest number in one year since the epidemic began. Three million die from AIDS in the same year. (-8)

G8 Evian Summit includes special focus on HIV/AIDS, new commitments to the Global Fund announced. (-9)

The William J. Clinton Presidential Foundation secures price reductions for HIV/AIDS drugs from generic manufacturers, to benefit developing nations. (-9)

"3 by 5" Initiative announced by World Health Organization, to bring treatment to 3 million people by 2005. (-9)

Activists express reservations about a provision that gives abstinence programs a third of USAID's prevention funding. (-9)

President Bush announces PEFAR, , the President's Emergency Plan for AIDS Relief, during the State of the Union Address; PEPFAR is a five-year, $15 billion initiative to address HIV/AIDS, tuberculosis, and malaria primarily in hard hit countries. (-9)

2004

A vaccine for AIDS is still years away, warns the IAVI. Less than 3% of all money devoted to AIDS goes towards developing a vaccine for the disease. (-8)

HIV blocking microbicides go on trial. The vaginal creams may provide a powerful weapon against the spread of HIV. Animal studies show some prevent infection in up to 75% of cases. (-8)

A drug that stops the HIV virus from stitching itself into human chromosomes is found to fight AIDS in an animal study. In the face of emerging drug-resistant HIV strains, the find could offer a new approach. (-8)

UNAIDS launches The Global Coalition on Women and AIDS to raise the visibility of the epidemic's impact on women and girls around the world. (-9)

PEPFAR, President Bush's Emergency Plan for AIDS Relief, begins first round of funding. (-9)

The Global Fund to Fight AIDS, Tuberculosis, and Malaria holds first ever "Partnership Forum", in Bangkok, Thailand. (-9)

2005

Around 40 million people are infected with AIDS worldwide. (-8)

A highly resistant strain of HIV linked to rapid progression to AIDS is identified in New York City, US. (-8)

Jesse Helms publishes an autobiography which outlines his changed stance on HIV/AIDS. (-9)

THE ECONOMIST reports on September 8, 2005: "The Global Fund estimates that it needs $7.1 billion from donors to fund projects in 2006 and 2007. At its "replenishment" conference this week in London, though, it received pledges totalling $3.7 billion. The fund reckons this is just enough cash to fill this year's shortfall of roughly $350m, and to pay for the renewal of projects already under way. What it does not allow, however, are any new projects over the next two years—unless more money is forthcoming." (-9)

Ranbaxy becomes first Indian drug manufacturer to gain U.S. Food and Drug Administration approval to produce generic antiretroviral for PEPFAR. (-9)

At World Economic Forum's Annual Meeting in Davos, Switzerland, priorities include a focus on addressing HIV/AIDS in Africa and other hard hit regions of the world. (-9)

The U.S. Food and Drug Administration grants "Tentative Approval to Generic AIDS Drug Regimen for Potential Purchase Under the President's Emergency Plan for AIDS Relief", marking first ever approval of an HIV drug regimen manufactured by a non-U.S.-based generic pharmaceutical company. (-9)

The World Health Organization, UNAIDS, the United States Government, and the Global Fund to Fight AIDS, Tuberculosis and Malaria announce results of joint efforts to increase the availability of antiretroviral drugs in developing countries. An estimated, 700,000 people had been reached by the end of 2004. (-9)

U.N. General Assembly High-Level Meeting on HIV/AIDS to review progress on targets set at 2001 U.N. General Assembly Special Session on HIV/AIDS (UNGASS). (-9)

The U.S Food and Drug Administration's Drugs Used in the Treatment of HIV Infection has added additional approved drugs:

July 12, 2006:
"Atripla" (brand name)- Efavirenz, Emtricitabine, Tenofovir DF (generic name) Class-Fixed Dose Combination (fixed dose combination tablets contain 2 or more anti-HIV medications that can be form 1 or more drug classes). Manufacturer- Bristol-Meyers Squibb, Gilead Sciences. (-17)

June 23, 2006:
"Prezita", TMC114 (brand name), Darunavir-Class-Protease Inhibitors (Pis) (Generic name). Manufacturer-Tibotec. (-17)

Successes in HIV Prevention
CDC's overarching HIV-prevention goal is to reduce the number of new HIV infections and to eliminate racial and ethnic disparities by the promotion of HIV counseling, testing, and referral and by encouraging HIV prevention among both persons living with HIV and those at high risk for contracting the virus (-18)

Prevention messages focused on both HIV-positive and HIV-negative persons.
Providing culturally and contextually appropriate messages is essential to help persons at risk avoid contracting HIV infection and to help those who are infected with HIV avoid transmitting the virus. Prevention messages also need to focus on the role of alcohol and drug abuse in HIV risk. Substance abuse (via injection drugs, alcohol, or methamphetamines) can facilitate risky behaviors among persons who might otherwise protect themselves and others from HIV. Preventing substance abuse and increasing access to substance-

abuse treatment are examples of effective interventions for reducing HIV transmission. (-18)

Special Issue of *MMWR*

HIV/AIDS remains a potentially deadly chronic disease. Prevention of HIV infection requires a continued commitment from persons at risk, persons infected, and society as a whole. Prevention efforts need to keep pace with a changing epidemic. Most importantly, younger generations, who might not remember the deadlier, early days of the epidemic, continually need to receive basic HIV-prevention messages. Twenty-five years after first reporting on AIDS, *MMWR* dedicates this issue to retrospectives on the epidemic, including the changing epidemiology of HIV/AIDS, the public health achievement in reducing perinatal transmission of HIV, and the evolution of measures to prevent HIV/AIDS. (-18)

Partnerships.

Eliminating HIV/AIDS in the United States cannot be achieved by any single agency or group, but will require public health partnerships comprising persons, communities, agencies, and the private sector. Strong partnerships are especially important to address stigma and discrimination and to promote greater acceptance of those living with HIV/AIDS. Religious and business communities and correctional and mental health services all need to be part of a national mobilization in the prevention of HIV transmission (*20*). Improved collaboration across government agencies is also required to provide a unified public health infrastructure dedicated to research, prevention, treatment, care, and rehabilitative services for persons affected by HIV/AIDS. (-19)

New prevention technologies.

Certain prevention technologies still under development, including pre-exposure prophylaxis, microbicides, and vaccines, are unlikely to provide full protection against HIV, might offer little or no protection against other STDs such as gonorrhea and chlamydia infections, and will not prevent unwanted pregnancies. Instead, new technologies are more likely to be incorporated into the spectrum of tools for comprehensive approaches to disease prevention. Effective behavior-change programs will still be needed to address possible behavioral disinhibition (i.e., continuing or returning to high-risk behaviors when one feels protected) among persons who receive these interventions. Prevention counseling that addresses informed choice and consent; the HIV-prevention behaviors of abstinence and delay of sexual debut, being monogamous, having fewer sex partners, and using condoms correctly and consistently; and other reproductive health needs (e.g., STD treatment and family planning) must be incorporated alongside these new prevention interventions. (-18)

This disease has connected all of us together. None of us are immune.

It is a human epidemic and it touches the heart of all of us.

CHAPTER 2

HIV/AIDS NUTRITION

Eating Defensively:
Food Safety Advice for Persons With AIDS

Bacteria and Food Poisoning

"It must have been something I ate!" How many times do people say this following about of nausea, upset stomach, cramps, diarrhea, or vomiting?

Indeed, these can be the symptoms of food poisoning--illness caused by eating food on which harmful bacteria have grown. The bacteria that cause food poisoning are difficult to detect by a food's appearance, taste or smell. But they can cause illness ranging from mild to very severe and even life-threatening. The human body ordinarily is well-equipped to deal with these bacteria, but individuals with weakened immune systems--such as those with acquired immune deficiency syndrome (AIDS) and those infected with the human immunodefiency virus (HIV)--can be far greater risk of serious illness. Because of their weakened immune systems, these individuals are more susceptible to contracting a food borne illness. Once contracted, these infections, with their severe vomiting and diarrhea, can be difficult to treat and they can come back again and again. This can further weaken the immune system and hasten the progression of HIV infection and be fatal for person with AIDS. (-13)

Why Do Bacteria Endanger People with AIDS?

When the AIDS virus damages or destroys the body's immune system, the person becomes more vulnerable to infection by food borne bacteria and other pathogens. For example, the common pneumonia, which is caused by a bacterial infection of the lungs, can occur in any individual but occurs much more frequently in persons with AIDS. In addition, when pneumonia strikes a person with AIDS, it causes a more severe illness and is thus more dangerous. (-14)

Persons with Acquired Immunodeficiency Syndrome (AIDS) are susceptible to many types of infection including illness from food borne pathogens. They are at higher risk than are otherwise healthy individuals for severe illness or death. Affected persons must be especially vigilant when handling and cooking foods. The recommendations provided here are designed to help prevent bacterial food borne illness. (-14)

What Types of Food borne Bacteria are of Particular Concern to Persons with AIDS?

Certain types of food borne illness are caused by bacteria which can grow on food. The bacteria can infect humans when the food is improperly handled or inadequately cooked. As with many other types of infections, persons with AIDS are at higher risk for developing severe illness or dying from these illnesses. Three types of bacteria are of particular concern for persons with AIDS: *Salmonella*, *Campylobacter jejuni*, and *Listeria monocytogenes*. (-14)

Salmonella bacteria are the most common cause of foodborne illness. The bacteria are commonly found on raw or undercooked meats (especially poultry) and can be found in eggs even before they are cracked open. Salmonellosis can affect anyone, but occurs almost 100 times more frequently in persons with AIDS than in otherwise healthy persons. Furthermore, *Salmonella* infections, which occur in persons with AIDS, can be particularly difficult to treat and are more likely to lead to serious complications. (-14)

Salmonellosis is the illness that can develop from eating foods containing Salmonella bacteria. It is characterized by flu-like symptoms, possibly accompanied by nausea, vomiting, abdominal cramps, and diarrhea. Symptoms can develop 6 to 48 hours after exposure and last up to a week. Foods most often associated with salmonellosis include raw or undercooked meat, poultry, fish, and eggs. (-13)

Illness from *Campylobacter jejuni* is also caused by a bacteria that can sometimes be found on food, especially raw poultry. This illness occurs about 35 times more frequently in persons with AIDS than in otherwise healthy persons. Many persons contract this form of food poisoning by improperly handling or cooking poultry. Raw milk and contaminated drinking water can also be sources of *Campylobacter.* (-14)

The symptoms of Campylobacter infection (campylobacteriosis) include acute abdominal pain, diarrhea (which can be watery and contain blood), nausea, headache, muscle pain, and fever. Symptoms can begin 2 to 5 days after eating contaminated food and generally lasts 7 to 10 days. Campylobacter bacteria are most commonly found in raw or undercooked poultry, unpasteurized milk, and non-chlorinated water. (-13)

Listeriosis

is caused by *Listeria monocytogenes* which can be found on many different types of food. *Listeria* infections are much more common in persons with AIDS than healthy people. *Listeria* infections in AIDS patients are usually severe and are often fatal. *Listeria monocytogenes* can be acquired from a variety of foods including soft cheeses that are unpasteurized and some ready-to-eat foods such as hot dogs or deli meats. (-14)

Listeriosis, the disease caused by Listeria, is characterized by flu-like symptoms of chills, fever and headache, sometimes accompanied by nausea and vomiting. These early symptoms can appear 2 to 30 days after exposure and can be followed by bacteremia (a bloodstream infection), meningitis (an inflammation of the membranes covering the spinal cord and brain), or encephalitis (an inflammation of the membranes of the brain itself). Foods found to contain Listeria are unpasteurized milk and cheeses, raw or undercooked meat, poultry, and fish. (-13)

How Can Persons with AIDS Prevent Food borne Illness?

Food must be handled safely at every stage from purchase through consumption. Critical points are transporting perishable foods home from the store immediately; prompt, safe storage; thorough cooking to destroy bacteria and other pathogens; and prompt refrigeration of leftovers. (-14)

Since most foodborne illnesses result from improper handling of food, person with AIDS or HIV infection can help themselves by following basic food safety guidelines. Applying these guidelines when buying, preparing and storing food, along with having a basic knowledge of the most common harmful bacteria and the foods on which they are found or can grow, can allow persons with AIDS to eat defensively while choosing a nutritious diet. (-13)

People cannot get AIDS from food. The food safety advice in this brochure is intended to help persons with HIV infection to reduce the risk of food poisoning, thereby avoiding an illness that could worsen their condition or even cause death. While many kinds of bacteria can cause food poisoning, three are the most prevalent threat to persons with AIDS and HIV infections. These are: Campylobacter, Listeria and Salmonella. (-13)

Shopping for Food

How to Shop Safely for Perishable FoodWhen shopping for raw and cooked perishable foods, be sure the food is being stored at a safe temperature in the store. Don't select perishable food from a non-refrigerated aisle display. Never choose packages which are torn or leaking. To guard against cross-contamination, put raw meat and poultry into a plastic bag so meat juices won't drip on other foods, such as lettuce and fruit that will be eaten raw. **Put refrigerated or frozen items in the shopping cart last, and take food home immediately**. (-14)

Deli Foods

When ordering food from the deli department, be sure the clerk washes his hands between handling raw and cooked items, or puts on new plastic gloves. Don't buy cooked ready-to-eat items which are touching raw items or are displayed in the same case. Although the risk associated with foods from deli counters is relatively low, persons at risk may choose to avoid these foods or thoroughly reheat luncheon meats and hot dogs before eating. (-14)

Shelf-Stable Foods

Don't purchase cans that are dented, leaking, or bulging; food in cracked glass jars; or food in torn packaging. Tamper-resistant safety seals should be intact. Safety buttons on metal lids should be down and should not move or make a clicking noise when pushed. (-14)Although product dating is not required by Federal regulations, observe any "use-by" dates found on products. **Do not use if beyond expiration date!** Follow carefully the handling and preparation instructions on product labels to ensure top quality and safety. (-14)For persons with AIDS, it is especially important to read food labels to select foods that pose the least risk of food poisoning. For example, all milk and cheese products should have the word "pasteurized" on the label. Products that contain any raw or undercooked meat or dairy products should be avoided, as well as products with a "sell by" or "best used by" date that has passed. (-13)

It is a good idea to put packaged meat, poultry or fish into plastic bag before placing it in the shopping cart. This prevents drippings from coming in contact with other foods and thus reduces the risks of cross-contamination--bacteria from one food contaminating another food. (-13)

The sale of food products with damaged packaging, the unsafe displaying of products (such as cooked shrimp on the same bed of ice as raw seafood), workers with poor personal hygiene, and unsanitary store conditions can add to the risk of food borne illness. Not only should consumers avoid purchasing food products sold under such conditions, but the conditions should be reported to local health authorities. (-13)

After shopping, get chilled and frozen foods into refrigerator or freezer as soon as possible. Storing them in a warm car or office or even just carrying them around for a couple of hours can raise the foods' temperature enough to allow bacteria to grow. (-13)

At Home
Food Storage
Immediately refrigerate or freeze perishable foods after transporting them home. Use a refrigerator thermometer to be sure the refrigerator is cooling to 40 °F or below; the freezer should be at 0 °F. (-14)

Refrigerator.
Make sure thawing juices from meat and poultry do not drip on other foods. Leave eggs in their carton for storage and don't place them in the door of the refrigerator. Keep the refrigerator clean. Store ground meat, poultry, and fish up to 1 or 2 days; other red meats, 3 to 5 days. After cooking, use within 3 to 4 days, or freeze for longer storage. (-14)

Freezer.
Food stored constantly at 0 °F will always be safe. Only the quality suffers with lengthy storage. It is of no concern if a product date expires while the product is frozen. Freezing keeps food safe by preventing the growth of microorganisms that cause both food spoilage and food borne illness. Once thawed, however, these microbes can again become active, so handle thawed items as any perishable food. (-14)

Pantry
Store canned foods and other shelf stable products in a cool, dry place. Never put them above the stove, under the sink, in a damp garage or basement, or any place exposed to high or low temperature

extremes. Store high acid foods such as tomatoes and other fruit up to 18 months; low acid foods such as meat and vegetables, 2 to 5 years. (-14)

Food Handling At Home

Foodborne illness can be caused by improper food handling or preparation in the home. Wash, utensils, can openers, cutting boards, and countertops in hot, soapy water before and after coming in contact with raw meat, poultry, or fish. Wash kitchen towels and cloths often in hot water in a washing machine. Wash hands with soap and warm water before and after handling food, and after using the bathroom, changing diapers, or handling pets. (-14)

Most cases of food poisoning are caused by improper food handling or preparation in the home. Keeping shelves, counter tops, refrigerators, freezers, utensils, sponges, and towels clean is one of the best ways to prevent bacterial contamination of food at home. It is especially important to wash all utensils and your hands with soap and hot water after handling one food and before handling another. This helps prevent cross-contamination in which, for example bacteria in raw meat could be transferred to other foods, such as salads or vegetables. For the same reason, wooden cutting boards should not be used for cutting raw meat, poultry or fish. Plastic boards are easier to clean and sanitize. Fresh fruits and vegetables should be thoroughly washed with water and refrigerated to reduce spoilage. the temperature in a refrigerator should be maintained at or below 40 deg F and food should be stored in covered containers. (-13)

Properly cooking food is another important guard against food poisoning. Heat kills bacteria. Most cookbooks give appropriate cooking times and temperature for different foods. A meat thermometer should be used to ensure complete cooking. Cook red meat until it is well done and poultry until the juices run clear. Thoroughly reheat leftovers (165 deg F).

Never eat raw eggs or foods that contain them. Pasteurized eggs should be used in place of shell eggs when making homemade ice cream, eggnog and mayonnaise. If you can't obtain pasteurized eggs, then you must omit the egg ingredient when making homemade ice cream. When cooking eggs, make sure that the yolk and white are firm, not runny. Here are cooking times and temperatures:

- Scrambled-1 minute at medium stove top setting (250 deg F for electric frying pans).
- Sunnyside-7 minutes at medium setting (250 deg F) or cook covered 4 minutes at 250 deg F.
- Fried, over easy-3 minutes at medium setting (250 deg F) on one side, then turn and fry for another minute on the other side.
- Poached-5 minutes in boiling water.
- Boiled-7 minutes in boiling water.

Microwave cooking requires special precautions. Most microwave recipes include a "standing time" after the cooking period to ensure that a proper temperature is reached throughout the food. Also, many microwave dishes must be removed from the oven and stirred from time to time-again, ensuring thorough cooking. It is particularly important to heat pre-cooked foods or leftovers thoroughly, whether in a microwave or conventional oven. (-13)

Eating Out
Many cases of foodborne illness are caused by restaurant, take-out, and deli-prepared foods. People at risk should avoid the same foods when eating out as they would at home. Meat, poultry, and fish should be ordered well done; if the food arrives undercooked, it should be sent back. (-14)

Cutting Boards
Research shows that nonporous surfaces, such as plastic, marble, tempered glass, and pyroceramic are easier to clean than wood. Wood surfaces are considered porous.Regardless of the type of cutting board you prefer, wood or a nonporous surface, consider using one for fresh produce and a separate one for raw meat, poultry, and

seafood. This will prevent bacteria on a cutting board that is used for raw meat, poultry, or seafood from cross-contaminating a food that requires no further cooking. (-14)Cutting boards need to be maintained and monitored for cleanliness. They should be washed with hot, soapy water or placed in the dishwasher. Solid hardwood cutting boards are dishwasher safe; however, wood laminates should not be washed in the dishwasher. (-14)After thoroughly washing your cutting board, you can sanitize it with a solution of 1 tablespoon of unscented, liquid chlorine bleach in 1 gallon of water. Once cutting boards of any type become excessively worn or develop hard-to-clean grooves, they should be discarded. (-14)

Restaurants, like grocery stores, are required to follow sanitation guideline established by state and local health departments to ensure cleanliness and good hygiene. Persons with AIDS need to avoid the same foods in restaurants that they would at home. Always order food well-done; if it served medium to rare, send it back. A good way to determine doneness is to cut into the center of a steak, hamburger, or other piece of meat. If it is the least bit pink or bloody, it needs more cooking. Fish should be flaky, not rubbery, when cut. (-13)

Order fried eggs cooked on both sides instead of sunny side up, and avoid scrambled eggs that look runny. Caesar salad should also be avoided since it contains raw eggs. If unsure about the ingredients in a particular dish, ask before ordering. (-13)

Raw seafood poses a serious risk of food poisoning for persons with AIDS. Raw shellfish, like raw meat and poultry, should be assumed to harbor harmful bacteria. Oysters on the half shell, raw clams, sushi and sashimi should not be eaten. Lightly steamed seafood, such as mussels and snails, should be avoided. (-13)

Cooking Food Safely
Do not eat raw or undercooked meat, poultry, fish, or eggs. For people with AIDS, the most important thing is to **use a food thermometer to be sure foods have reached a safe minimum internal**

temperature. (-14) Cook foods to the following safe minimum internal temperatures as measured with a food thermometer:

- Beef, veal, and lamb steaks, roasts, and chops may be cooked to 145 °F.
- All cuts of pork to 160 °F.
- Ground beef, veal and lamb to 160 °F.
- Egg dishes, casseroles to 160 °F.
- Leftovers to 165 °F.
- Stuffed poultry is not recommended. Cook stuffing separately to 165 °F.
- All poultry should reach a safe minimum internal temperature of 165 °F. (-14)

When reheating foods in the microwave, cover and rotate or stir foods once or twice during cooking and check the food in several spots with a food thermometer. (-14)

Safe Handling of Leftovers

Bacteria begin to multiply rapidly in the "danger zone" between 40 °F (recommended refrigerator temperature) and 140 °F. Therefore, bacteria on food left out at room temperature will become unsafe in a matter of hours. Refrigerate leftovers at 40 °F or below or freeze (0 °F) as soon as possible. **Never leave perishable food out of refrigeration longer than 2 hours, 1 hour in air temperatures above 90 °F.** (-14)

Divide leftovers into shallow containers. This encourages rapid, even cooling. Cover with airtight lids or enclose in plastic wraps or aluminum foil. Use leftovers within 3 to 4 days. (-14)

Safe Reheating of Leftovers

Even though foods may have been safely cooked, bacteria from the air or people's hands can contaminate the leftovers. Always reheat leftovers thoroughly in a conventional or microwave oven or on the stove top. When reheating foods in the microwave, cover and rotate or stir foods once or twice during cooking. Always test reheated leftovers in several places with a food thermometer to be sure they reach 165 °F throughout. The food should be steaming hot. (-14)

Traveling Abroad

Persons with AIDS should take additional precautions when traveling abroad. Boil all water. Drink only canned or carbonated bottled drinks or use beverages and ice made with boiled water. Avoid uncooked vegetables and salads. All fruit should be peeled. All foods should be cooked thoroughly and eaten while still hot. (-14)

Not all countries have the same high standards of hygiene and sanitation as the United States, so persons with AIDS should take additional precautions when traveling abroad.

Boil all water before drinking. Drink only beverages made with boiled water or canned or carbonated bottled drinks. Ice, too, should be made only from boiled water. Avoid uncooked vegetables and salads. All fruit should be peeled. Eat cooked foods while they are still hot. (-13)

A good rule of thumb is "Boil it, cook it, peel it, or forget it." (-13)

While food poisoning can usually be treated with rest and plenty fluids until solid food can be eaten again, persons with AIDS or HIV infection may experience prolonged and more serious symptoms requiring a doctor's care. (-13)

If a consumer or doctor believes that an attack of food poisoning was related to a particular food or restaurant, the local health department or the Food and Drug Administration should be contacted. Reporting the incident to health officials can help others avoid serious illness. The telephone number for FDA's Emergency Operations Branch is 301-443-1240 (this number is staffed 24 hours a day). (-13)

These food safety guidelines for persons with AIDS and HIV infection are no different than those recommended for anyone. But, in the case of persons with AIDS or HIV infection, contaminated food can have more serious consequences. (-13)

There are other high-risk groups--such as cancer patients, diabetics, transplant recipients, infants, pregnant women, and the elderly--who should also give special attention to those guidelines. For individuals in these high-risk groups, maintaining a nutritious diet is of great importance. Cooking and eating defensively need not interfere with a nutritious diet. But not being aware of the hazards and not taking appropriate steps to reduce the risk food poisoning can be life-threatening. (-13)

For additional food safety information about meat, poultry, or egg products, call the toll-free USDA Meat and Poultry Hotline at 1-888-674-6854; for the hearing-impaired (TTY) 1-800-256-7072. The Hotline is staffed by food safety experts weekdays from 10 a.m. to 4 p.m. Eastern time. Food safety recordings can be heard 24 hours a day using a touch-tone phone. (-14)

Sources:

(-13) U. S. Food and Drug Administration FDA Brochure: 1992 http://www.cfsan.fda.gov/~dms/aidseat.html

(-14) United States Department of Agriculture Food Safety and Inspection Service http://www.fsis.usda.gov/Fact Sheets/ Food Safety for Persons with AIDS/index.asp

CHAPTER 3

TESTIMONY

Myself

In composing my personal journal writings, I would like present to you, a look at the events leading to the choices, and decisions I've made in my life. I hope my testimony, enables you to make meaning out of my experience, and to see the consequences of my actions, may it be bad or good. My destiny, was structured based on each choice I made.

The year was 1984: Born and raised in a middle class family, one of five children in Brooklyn NY. I was nineteen years, old just starting my life. Family and friends surrounded my life. Unfortunately, everything slowly came apart. I was ALANON.

February 12, 1984: Was the day my mother died of Cancer. It was a very difficult time for all of us. My mother, was a warm loving, spiritual, caring woman, however, deeply troubled. She was, an alcoholic. She eventually, stopped daily drinking, and became a holiday drinker. Most of our family holidays were spent, watching mom with a flashlight dancing around the house, with her black sunglasses on at night. She always had a beer, and a cigarette in her hand. It was very bizarre watching mom, be "house mom", throughout the year, then party mom during the holidays. Apparently, I was not aware, of how dysfunctional this was in which, I found out later on. Living in our two-family home was, my grandfather and uncle, which also were alcoholics. My mother, was a very lonely, depressed, insecure woman, even-though my father was present. She never searched for professional help. Professional help would mean, you had a problem or were unstable. How can an unstable mother, care for her five children? Where I come from, it was unheard of. Personal problems, were left in your closet of dark secrets untold. I believe, Cancer is an inward growth. Emotions unexpressed, and suppressed. I think given the opportunity of counseling, my mother would be alive today.

During her life as, "house mom", she secluded herself. Never, leaving the home, or conversing with people.

Neither, was I allowed to have friends visit the home. Mom, spent much of her time, with her compulsion for cleaning and taking care of the immediate family, that's it. My memories of mom, were nothing but nurturing, and loving, filled with compassion. These traits developed me to the person, I am today.

With the passing of my mother, things began to change. My father, moved out of the home. Grandma, Grandpa, and Uncle Mike died between 1985 and 1987.

All my brothers and sisters, scattered, and relocated to different parts of the city.

At nineteen years old, I was immediately faced to become independent. I obtained my first apartment, with a bed, a bureau and rent for a month. I was fresh out of High School. Unfortunately for me, college was not an option.

My life as an adult, had arrived. Being an adult, gave me so much freedom but at price. With my newfound freedom, I was in nightclubs 3 times a week. I found myself, drinking, and smoking on every occasion. It seemed, that everyone was doing the same thing. It didn't seem, unusual to me. I was also attractive, which didn't hurt the situation. I was free. Free with no restrictions, and no supervision. You would think being nineteen years old, I would be a pretty responsible adult, but I was a still a naïve little girl, in a woman's body. Late 1984, I had my first serious relationship. He was, 27 years old. Why, in the world, would a nineteen year old girl want with a 27 year old man? All I knew, was how he was so attentive to my needs, at least, that's how I seen it. I met him in NY, rushing to catch the train. He was a train conductor, for the New York City Transit Authority. Now being independent, and wanting to be loved, I allowed him into my life, at a very vulnerable time. On the contrary, a relationship is no way to fill unfulfilled needs. There is a big price to pay for instant gratification. We dated for several months, and within those months, I noticed disturbing behaviors. We had an accident in his car, when he blacked out. He would nod, like he was falling asleep right in the middle of a conversation. It seemed, at times he was dazed and confused.

I never encountered, anyone behave like this before. I was hesitant, to ask him if there was something wrong. I wasn't concerned, as long as he paid attention, and loved me. That was all that mattered. (Yeah right).

The relationship became intimate, and I never practiced safe sex.

Why should I?

Let me tell you the things I said:

Nothing will happen to me!

I can tell, by the way a person looks!

Bad things happen to bad people, in bad neighborhoods!

I am a good person, in a good neighborhood, knowing good people!

I had so many misconceptions. How lost, and blind, I really was. The absence of supervision, and wisdom from my parents, resulted in my lack of knowledge. My parents, never taught education at home, not to mention the topic of sex. I know my parents had sex, for there would not have been so many siblings. GOD forbid, they talk to us. My oldest brother, wasn't spoken to, (for he now has seven children all starting at the age of 15). That was just one, of the many topics you did not talk about. For my need for love, and security was so great, that I thought I was untouchable.

The relationship was having some difficulty, and my partner became physically abusive. He had hit me a few times, stole money from me, lied and cheated, but, I loved him.

I continued this relationship for a few years, but I didn't understand why. I actually thought, I deserved to pay that price, for his love, and attention. My mother, self sacrificed her life for her husband, and family, why shouldn't I. A decision, which turned out to be abusive, was the price I paid for love. My friends, finally convinced me to stop the madness, and abuse.

To my surprise, I was out of control. I really did not see, that this was not a functional relationship. As a matter of fact, I didn't think anything was wrong. He has a few problems, everyone does. I'm unique, I have the patience to have a relationship like this (oh brother).

After steeling my rent money, and not wanting to lose my apartment, and endure further physical abuse, I reluctantly, broke my relationship with my 27-year old boyfriend. I was unable, to sever my involvement with him.

I so deeply loved him, for reasons I could not understand. I became withdrawn, and very depressed. After the breakup, I never heard, or seen him again.

1986, I returned to the dating scene at some of my favorite hot spots in Brooklyn NY. Once again, much attention was spent trying to fill my empty void. It was an obsession. I was introduced by a friend, to one of the bartenders of the bar. One conversation led to another. Before you know, it I was in a relationship again. The void was filled!

My new boyfriend, was nothing like my previous boyfriend. He was smart, fun, kind, and honest. He was a real nice guy. How boring. Could you believe, I finally was dating a nice guy, and I found him not to be satisfying, (go Figure). I seemed to enjoy drama, and chaos. Regardless of how I felt, I continued to date him even though he wasn't a challenge to me.

On February 14, 1987: My boyfriend after work, arrived to speak to me about my ex boyfriend, (the one who was the Transit worker, and that I haven't heard from since the breakup). He knew a little bit about him, due to previous conversations. They also had encounters.

My boyfriend sat me down, and handed me a stuffed animal, a card for Valentine's Day. I was so touched. However, after handing me the gift, he held my hand, and said to me, I have very serious information concerning us. One of the employees at the bar, informed me that your ex-boyfriend died of AIDS. I immediately, became quiet. I became totally numb, from head to toe. I felt the energy escape from my body. I asked my boyfriend to repeat what he had said, and he replied the same information. Once again, I was silent. This can't be true.

Yet this time, I felt this black cloud come over me. I began to feel, all kinds of emotions. I was sad, but also fearful. I asked myself why is he telling me this. Does he think? Can I? Is it possible? How could this happen? I should have known. What does this all mean? My mind was racing.

I was trying to rationalize, and process the information, I had received. I became sick, and nervous. My hands were shaking. I began to cry. After composing myself, my boyfriend, suggested I try to get in contact with my ex-boyfriends parents, to confirm the information. We talked for a little while.

He recommended, we go get tested for HIV. I was terrified. I couldn't even think of it. I told him, let me find out if this information is true or not. Under the circumstances, I proceeded to approach the situation, with hope. I was so upset, and asked my boyfriend to give me some time to sort this out. I decided to send him home, and get back to him once I had some information.

The evening of February 14, 1987: I called the home of my ex-boyfriends parents. I dial, the phone rings, his mother answers. Hi this is V. I know we haven't spoken since (ex-boyfriend), and I broke-up. However, I have disturbing information I need to speak with you about. Rumor has it that, (ex-boyfriend), had died of AIDS. Is this true? There was silence on the other end of the phone. My heart was pounding, for I knew it was true. She kindly replied come to the house, so we can talk. Without saying a word, she had said all. I needed to know. Once again, my body went numb.

I kept my feelings, and thoughts to myself. I traveled by train, to the home of my ex-boyfriends parents. As I was riding the train, it seemed like eternity to get there. Each minute seemed like hours. I couldn't comprehend, if I was coming or going. I was flooded with emotions. As the train approached my stop, I felt the pounding of my steps, up my legs, traveling up until I felt pulsations in my ears as I walked off the train. I will never, forget the feelings. I walked through the streets, like I was in slow motion. I was lifeless. I tried to compose myself, just a few more blocks. At last, I finally arrived to the home.

I rang the bell, she answered, and let me in. I examined her face, to see if there were signs that would give me any clues.

She looked very tired. I prepare myself for the news. She loving seated me, and sat down beside me. I spoke to her in a very soft voice, is it true? Softly, she responded, yes. I fell apart. The tears began to roll down my face uncontrollably. My world, had fallen apart. She did her best to comfort me, but I was torn apart. I spent a good time with her, and the family, and she continued to inform me of the reasons why, he did not attempt to call me.

She shared with me, the severe suffering he endured. He also, went blind.

She had told me that he tried to call me once, but decided not to speak. She told me he had been using injection drugs, and contracted HIV, which turned into AIDS by needle sharing.

I had no idea, he was an intravenous drug user. All that time I spent with him, watching him act peculiar, all seemed to make sense now. I never thought, it was drugs. The pain, sorrow, fear, and anxiety overwhelmed me. My ex-boyfriend's parents, drove me home that evening. We said our good byes, and I proceeded into my apartment. I now, have to tell my boyfriend that the information is true.

The next morning, I called my boyfriend and told him I needed to speak to him. I haven't slept all night. I had such anxiety, and fear. I shared this information with my childhood friends, and roommates. They could not believe it. They looked at me, with such remorse.

They were also afraid for me. My girlfriends, and I talked, and cried while waiting for the arrival of my boyfriend. I was worried about him, as well as myself. What am I going to say? What are we going to do? What is everyone going to think? So many things were running through my mind. In the meantime, we comforted each other.

The bell rings. It was my boyfriend. I approach the door with such sorrow in my heart. This information, would totally change us forever.

I open the door. His blue eyes pieced me. I was unable to speak. My reaction to his presence, said it all. He walked into the apartment.

He proceeded to speak. We need to get tested right away.

Without words, I nodded, and agreed. We just stayed quietly together, and fell asleep.

Monday morning February 1987: my boyfriend and I, arrive at the doctor's office to take our HIV test. Each of us, was taken to a separate room, and was spoken to by the physician. The doctor asked me, why I wanted an HIV test, in which I had explained the information I had received. He was very sympathetic, and concerned. He consoled me on the results of a negative, or a positive test, and how long it would take to receive the results.

Unfortunately, there was not much hope at the time, if the results were positive. The only information the doctor could supply, was education, support, patience, and compassion. It must have been very hard for doctors in the 1980's, to be doctors, for there was nothing they could do to help the many people who currently had AIDS. My blood was drawn. I now, have to wait two weeks for the results. The waiting game begins.

For the next two weeks, I tried to keep myself busy. It was the longest two weeks of my life. I was playing the, "what if", game with myself. I started reflecting, on my behaviors that led me to where I am today. I was blaming myself, feeling dirty, and ashamed. Feeling so naïve, I became angry and upset. I began to blame others for this situation I was in.

My emotions were out of control. I had to try to keep it together. Day by day, hour after hour, the anxiety, and anticipation was building. I started bargaining with GOD. If GOD would spare me from this situation, I would do anything. So, with this hope, I was able to buy a day or two. However, the doubts would return. I was trying to keep myself as stable as possible, without anyone knowing. I found it so hard, to function in my everyday life, and yet I continued on. This was the first week.

The beginning of week two was even more extreme. The anxiety, and anticipation increased. I was unable, to control my emotions. I was unable, to concentrate. My work, was compromised. I did inform my employer of my situation, in which, they were very patient, and understanding with me during this difficult time. I was useless, to everyone.

I was a moving mummy. I didn't know, if I was coming or going. Each day, I proceeded like a robot. I went to work, ate very little, bargained with GOD, and went to sleep. I spoke to no one. I just, existed in the world. For the next two weeks, I waited for the answer to my destiny.

There was a day or two, where I would play mind games with myself. I would tell myself, that this is not happening. This is all, a bad dream. Nothing, is going to happen. All, will be fine. I would tell myself, everything, is going to be ok. I'm making a big deal, out of nothing.

This will not, happen to you. I was thinking of different reasons why, this could not happen to me. This was just temporary relief. My thoughts bounced, back and forth. from negative, to positive thoughts each, and everyday. Many people, tend to be "controlling" personalities, in which I happen to be. For a controlling person, to be so "out of control" is like torture.

I found out through this experience, that I am in control of nothing. During each day, my anxiety increases. By the end of week two, I was physically, mentally, and emotionally drained.

Friday February 1987: Today, is the day I would receive the HIV results. Would today, be the day where my roller coaster ride ends? Would this last two weeks just disappear? Would I wake up, from this nightmare? Or would this day, be the beginning of the end.

I managed, to go to work, continuing to control my emotions. I call the doctors office from my place of employment. I ask, to speak to the doctor.

The doctor, comes to the phone. I ask him, if the results arrived for my test. He responds, yes. At that moment, I just needed to know. I couldn't wait anymore. I start yelling at him, to give me the results. He responds, the results are POSITIVE for HIV antibodies. I drop the phone, fell to the floor, and wept uncontrollably.

As I sat on the floor, my employer, and supervisor rushed to my assistance.

They took me to one of the private offices. My employer, allowed me to express my feelings, and emotions. To my surprise, my employers were well prepared to deal with an employee with HIV. I thought, they were going to release me of my duties to the company, but they did not.

Today was a day, filled with uncertainty. Unquestionably, I can honestly say, today was the lowest day of my life. As I regained control of my emotions, sitting on the floor, I realized, it couldn't get any lower than this. For a moment, a feeling of peace came over me. I had to decide, whether I was going to fight, or give up. Did I have enough fight in me, to fight the good fight? I had to find a feasible method, to give it my best shot.

I didn't want to give up. I decided I wanted to live! Even-though, the results were grim, I wanted to try. This episode in my life, would be the beginning of my transformation, and my growing hope, and relationship with GOD.

My employers, continued to consol me. One of the supervisors, suggested I go get some professional help, and counseling on HIV and AIDS. They pointed out to me, the many people attending groups for support, during this difficult time. It's a support meeting, where people can express their feelings, fears, and personal experiences. It would be, a network of HIV/AIDS individuals, one helping each other. My supervisor, handed me a few phone numbers to a few locations, nearby the office. I was very fortunate, that my employers were so supportive, and understanding with my present situation. As you have read in the previous chapters, many people were not treated in the same manner. I became fearful. My life, was on a different path. I was walking into the unknown. I called, one of the support groups in the area. I had decided, to attend a support group.

That evening, my supervisor had drove me home. I told the news to my roommates. I don't suggest you tell people about anything personal about yourself until you yourself have accepted your situation. Upon telling the news to my roommates, I had mixed reactions. One of my room-mates, was a radiologist.

She understood the disease, for she had learned in her studies in radiology, the methods of transmission, and was well educated in the matter. On the other, hand my other roommate, was not as understanding.

She used the information as a conversation piece, in some of the bars in the neighborhood. So, what about my boyfriend, how did he react? As you know, he had also went for the HIV antibody test. Upon receiving my results, I had called my boyfriend. We discussed the results.

He was negative, for which, I was relieved. As for myself, I was concerned. What would this mean to us?

When discussing the results with each other, we realized that we were heading in different directions. We tried to work through the relationship. Unfortunately, the more people knew about my situation, the harder it was for my boyfriend, to deal with the stigma it had on me.

He did not want to be labeled in the same way. As a result, he broke away from the relationship. He made different excuses, in every encounter we had. This was the response of the people in my life and the people who knew about my situation. The news of my HIV status spread like wildfire.

Watch out!

Here she comes!

There's that girl with AIDS!

Don't go near her!

For ten years, I dealt with fear, anxiety, discrimination, stigma, and loneliness. I was no longer accepted, in my previous world. Many of my friends, no longer associated with me. Some of my so-called friends, would exclude me from their homes. They only invited me to outside catered events. They kept me at bay. I had to let go of my past life, and adapt to a new. I found my new life, through GOD, and my support groups.

March 1987: I attended my first HIV support group. I arrived to the support group room, and there was no one present. I entered the room wondering, what it was going to be like. What was I going to see? Would they judge me like other people? I entered, and took a seat in the middle of the room. In the room, there was a beautiful picture of cool waters flowing down a stream. As I gazed at the picture, I felt at peace. I knew, I was where I needed to be. Other people, finally arrived to attend the support group. They were regular everyday people, just like me.

I don't know what I expected, but I would have never known these people would have this disease. Nobody, would know by looking at me, that I had, HIV. We were newly diagnosed individuals with HIV, (a symptomatic: showing no symptoms of the disease). There were fifteen people who attended the meeting that day.

We all introduced ourselves. One cannot express, the long suffering, and sadness, and to find new found release. We shared painful experiences, as well as positive approaches on health, and nutritional options. We developed a caring family.

A place we felt safe, and secure. We developed meaningful friendships, and relationships.

We supported each other, through good times, and bad. I found a place, where I was accepted, and embraced. I was in a place, where I could me myself, a person living with HIV.

I continued to attend the HIV support group. I also started attending, an ALANON support group. ALANON, is a support group for children of alcoholics. As I attended this support group, much information reflected the fact, that I have developed many patterns, and habits of an alcoholic. These findings, helped me to restructure my mind to make healthier choices, better decisions, and a growing relationship with GOD's scriptures. This life change, would not happen over night. Through grace, and trust in GOD, because GOD is in control of our lives, and the tools I received attending group meetings, I was able to apply them to my life, making subtle changes daily. Transformation for me, was a gradual movement, and a decision to see things differently. I would like to emphasize, the importance of the decision I made to change. It took nineteen years, for me to develop my habits and behaviors. Therefore, it will take a while to correct them. I call it my daily mental workout. Time, must be vested in the work, (I will speak on this topic further in chapter 8). I continue to grow each, and everyday.

1987-1990: Where we first had fifteen people in our HIV support group, we now have four. Many of the members, had developed, and died of AIDS. It was a very sad time. I had attended many funerals. I attended funerals for other young people who had died in which the cause of death was not mentioned but I knew. The disease was all around us, and yet the four of us were still alive with no symptoms.

How blessed we were. During this time we continued to have faith and supported each other. We continued to fight. We continued to pray to GOD for guidance, healing and protection. We also continued to condition our minds to think positive thoughts. The main reason why I am here today, is because of my decision to have faith in GOD for my destiny, for his purpose, and will for my life. To control of my mind from negative habits, and thoughts,(mental control).

To eat well, take vitamins, herbal remedies for our immune system and exercise.

September 1, 1990: I married a friend, from my HIV support group. It seemed so much easier, to have a relationship with someone with the same situation. We had a lot in common. Eventhough, we were both HIV positive, we still needed to wear condoms. We needed to wear condoms so we would not re-:expose each other to the different strands of the virus, in which many people are not aware of.

February 1990: My husband and I, went on a ski trip. It was our second honeymoon. After our intimate moment, we discovered the condom we had used had torn.

What are we going to do now?

What if I get pregnant?

What if I do get pregnant and the baby gets HIV?

I thought we were being safe?

Would I have to abort?

Once again, I encounter another test of my faith.

Sure enough I was pregnant. It's bad enough I had HIV but now I am pregnant and would possibly pass the disease to my unborn child. I had to make a decision.

MY SECOND BIG TEST OF FAITH:

Despite what people may say, through studying, and reading my bible, and learning the word of GOD, I knew what my decision would be. I would keep my baby! There would be many obstacles, I would face. There was a 26% chance, that the baby would be exposed to the virus. Having a C-section would lower the percent to 15%.

So, I took that chance. During my pregnancy, I secluded myself, so that my family, and friends would not try to convince me to abort my child. Many people, would have thought it to be, a selfish move on my part. I believed, it would be a sin for me to make that decision, and that decision was not mine to make. I chose, to deal with the decision I made, and the consequences. I took good care of myself. I surrounded myself, with beautiful music, and read many books. In my third month of my pregnancy, I developed complications, in which bed rest was recommended. I recovered, and continued through the pregnancy. On my exact due date, I went into labor. Complications developed, and I was forced to have an emergency C-section, (which, happen to be a blessing in my situation). On November 1992: We were the proud parents of a baby girl. I would like to mention, she was negative for HIV antibodies. It also helped, having a C-section delivery because the baby was not exposed to blood, and fluids through the birth canal. What a miracle!!! How faithful GOD is!!! I had put all my faith in him and he was faithful!!!!

Once again, GOD had revealed to me his wonderful gifts, and goodness. I could have done what everyone thought I should do, but I did not. I used every ounce of my being, to be faithful and obedient to the decision of faith.

As a result, we were victorious. The price of our faith was the biggest blessing given, a healthy baby girl. The power of GOD can move mountains! All things are possible through GOD, and the blood shed from our Lord Jesus Christ. I happen to be a Christian, and GOD's Holy Spirit is alive and well inside me, guiding my every step.

I continue to be blessed with his many gifts each and everyday as you will read in my testimony. I share my GOD with you so you too can experience his power, strength and abilities in your life. As I continue with my story, you will see his tremendous influence in every aspect of my life. I hope in your continued reading of this book, you will find your way to GOD, and claim the blood of Jesus. Place all your worries, and concerns in his hands. Let GOD control your life, and do what Jesus would have done.

In return you will receive the rewards of his peace, love, blessings, gifts, goodness and his faithfulness to you.

As I continue feeding my mind, and soul with GOD's word, the enemy continues to test me. From 1992-1996 my marriage was in turmoil. We opened a new business, we had financial problems, and my husband began to drink. My husband, was an alcoholic, but discontinued when we met, and did not drink during the beginning of our marriage.

For some reason, the pressure was too much for him, the business, the baby etc. You are probably saying, why would I have a relationship with a former alcoholic? Good question. Remember, old habits still remained. Eventhough, I was learning, and attending support groups often, I still had old habits being transformed. I thought, I was strong enough to handle the relationship with the tools I learned. Subsequently, I wasn't. The relationship worsened, as months went on. Each day, he blamed me for every bad thing that happened. He began drinking excessively. He became jealous, of my attention given to the baby. He became irritated, when I associated with my family, so, I had stopped communications with them.

He was possessing total control of me. I stopped attending support groups. I attended to his needs. I was afraid, he would leave me alone, being HIV, unemployed and with a baby. I did what ever he asked. When I was compliant to his needs, he did not harass me. Day by day, he gained control over me, and I lost my identity. My life, did not belong to me anymore. It belonged to him. My life, was irrelevant. I was married now, I needed to change my ways. He wanted me to change to his ways. It was evident, that the situation was not going to change unless, I changed it.

In 1996: Under the influence of alcohol and psychotropic drugs, my husband approached my cousin and I, with a 357- magnum revolver. The insanity, had to come to an end. Fortunately, my cousin was able to retrieve the gun from his hand. Unfortunately for my husband, the police arrived and placed him under arrest for attempted murder. He served eight months in a penitentiary workforce program. Once again I was alone.

This time, it was different. Something inside of me had changed. As a result of this situation, I would have the time to find myself again, to start over. I was ready to give it a go.

While my husband was in the penitentiary, I began a relationship with GOD. I had always believed in GOD, and I knew Jesus sacrificed his life for me, but I never realized that you could have a relationship with him. I didn't even know how to pray. I was raised Catholic, and only knew the prayer's that I was taught. I began, by talking to him as if I was talking to a friend. At first, it seemed weird to me. I felt like a crazy person talking to air. How wrong I was! Each day turned into weeks, weeks into months. I followed the steps of Jesus, the faith of Job, the wisdom of David, and the boldness of Aaron and Moses, (My mentor's from the Bible). I don't believe, anyone can live a happy, peaceful, joyous, secure life without him.

A year had passed, and my husband was released for the penitentiary. He called me, and pleaded with me to take him back, and give him one more chance. I didn't know what to do. With the help of GOD, I was able to get back on my feet again. I was so abused. I am a GOD fearing woman. I know, how GOD feels about marriage vows. I did not want to displease him. I prayed to GOD, for strength. I asked GOD, to allow me to give him one more chance. I know, GOD does not want me to suffer, however, I will give my husband one more chance. I was a stronger woman now. I would put all my trust in GOD.

It took my husband three weeks to turn back to his old self again. I did not want to become a statistic of other battered women, so, I took immediate action.

I removed him from my premises, and filed an order of protection. Months later I filed for divorce.

I did it!! June 1996 my divorce was final, and I was free.

In conclusion, and being a true witness to this testimony, I have been through many trials, and tribulations. For my life was spared by GOD. I made a decision, and chose to dedicate the rest of my life to a relationship, and service to him. Each day I serve him, the better my life becomes. Each day, I am blessed with his wonderful gifts. He has blessed me, with a new husband. Like Abraham, (from the Bible) with the sale of our home from NY, my husband and I, were able to relocate and buy a home in Florida without having a mortgage payment. Several months later, I was led to volunteer for a not for profit HIV/AIDS organization, nearby my home, in which I still serve.

Joyce Meyer, whom I adore, says "we need to be in the world, not of the world".

In order to make a difference, we need to be different, and become leaders. I am just a servant, sharing the choices, and decisions that have worked in my life. I understand, many people have had bad experiences in Churches, but, I am not telling you to go to Church or not go to Church. However, we need Church to fellowship, and to strengthen us. I also know, the Church lives in us! Each one of us, can be the truth, the way, and the light. We need to live holy lives.

GOD knows, we are not perfect. GOD cares, about the quality of your life right now! He wants you to live in the light-fearlessly, abundantly, immeasurably. We can meet GOD, wherever we are in our lives. We need to surrender, and seek GOD. To seek GOD, is through his word, the Bible. For my GOD, is a loving GOD. He has taught me, the only way out is going through the trial. I hope I can convince you, to do the same. Seek GOD first, for who he is. Ask yourself, what kind of an impact I would like to have in the world.

Enjoying everyday life, and appreciating all the beauty around, and knowing how it came to be. Quality time spent with family, Church members, and friends.

To see the sunrise and the sunset and completing a day well lived. Surround yourself with inspirational music. To be content everyday and thankful for blessings and gifts. During all situations be positive and motivated.

Apply, "The fruits of the Spirit" to your life, (love, joy, peace, patience, kindness, goodness, faithfulness, gentleness, and self-control). To forget about oneself and to help, and assist others in need. To offer others hope, love, encouragement, and happiness as well. To go to work, and to love what you do!! To allow us time to meditate, and to reflect. Become obedient, and well balanced in all that we do. Believe that GOD, has a plan for your life. Everything we do can be part of GOD's plan. When we believe, it's just the beginning. Most of all, to know whom our guiding light, and strength comes from being a Christian, and believing in our Father GOD, through Jesus Christ.

"You will know them by their fruit"
(Mat 7:20) KJV

Are you weary and burdened?
Ask "He will give you rest"
(Mat 11:28) KJV

Do you need a new outlook on life?
Seek. He will "give you a new heart and put a new spirit in you"
(Ezekiel 36:26) KJV

Do you long for direction?
Knock. "He will give you another Counselor to be with you forever"
(John 14:16) KJV

Be children of light and avoid darkness in your life
"Let your light shine"
(Mat 5:16) KJV

"Continue to work out your salvation with fear and trembling, for it is GOD, who works in you to will and to act according to his good purpose"
(Phil 2:12, 13) KJV

"I am the light of the world. Whoever follows me will never walk in darkness, but will have the light of life"
(John 8:12) KJV

"Ask and it will be given to you; seek and you will find; knock and the door will be opened to you"
(Luke 11:19) KJV

This is the meaning of life, to me.
V.Perez

GOD is faithful!

CHAPTER 4

WHAT YOU DON'T KNOW CAN HURT YOU

This is a very important chapter for all individuals, communities, young or old, men or female, ill or healthy having active sex lives.

I graciously thank, Mr. James R. Hinson, Operations, Management and Consultant, and Raj Hiralal, of the Orange County Health Department for his presentation on July 2006 series workshop and for the use of this valuable information provided in this chapter.

In this chapter, you will find life saving and crucial information to your over all wellness.

Please note:
Some pages many be graphic in nature.

Sexually Transmitted Disease & You

Raj Hiralal
Jim Hinson

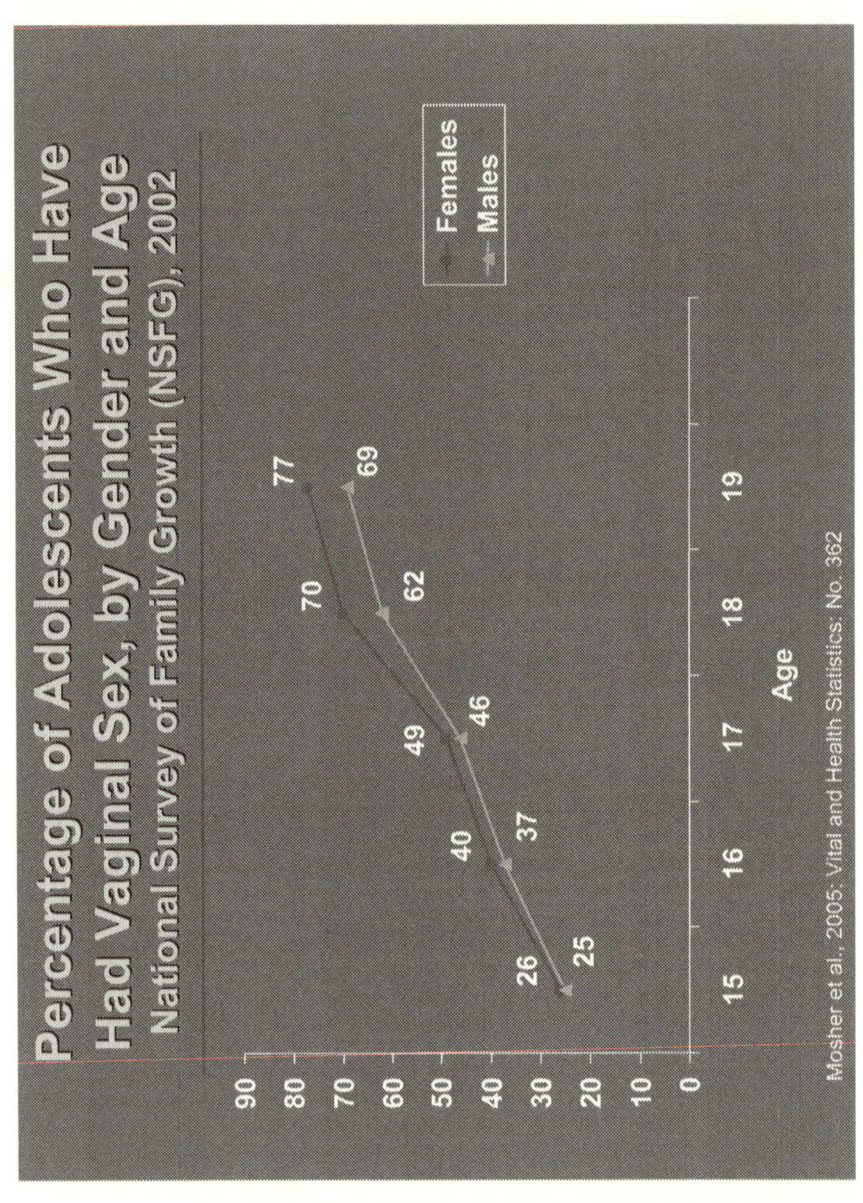

Percentage of Adolescents Who Have Had Vaginal Sex, by Gender and Age
National Survey of Family Growth (NSFG), 2002

Females
Males

77
70
69
62
49
46
40
37
26
25

Age

15 16 17 18 19

90 80 70 60 50 40 30 20 10 0

Mosher et al., 2005: Vital and Health Statistics: No. 362

Common STD's

- **Gonorrhea**
- **Chlamydia**
- **Syphilis**
- **Herpes**
- **Genital Warts (HPV)**
- **Hepatitis A, B & C**
- **HIV**

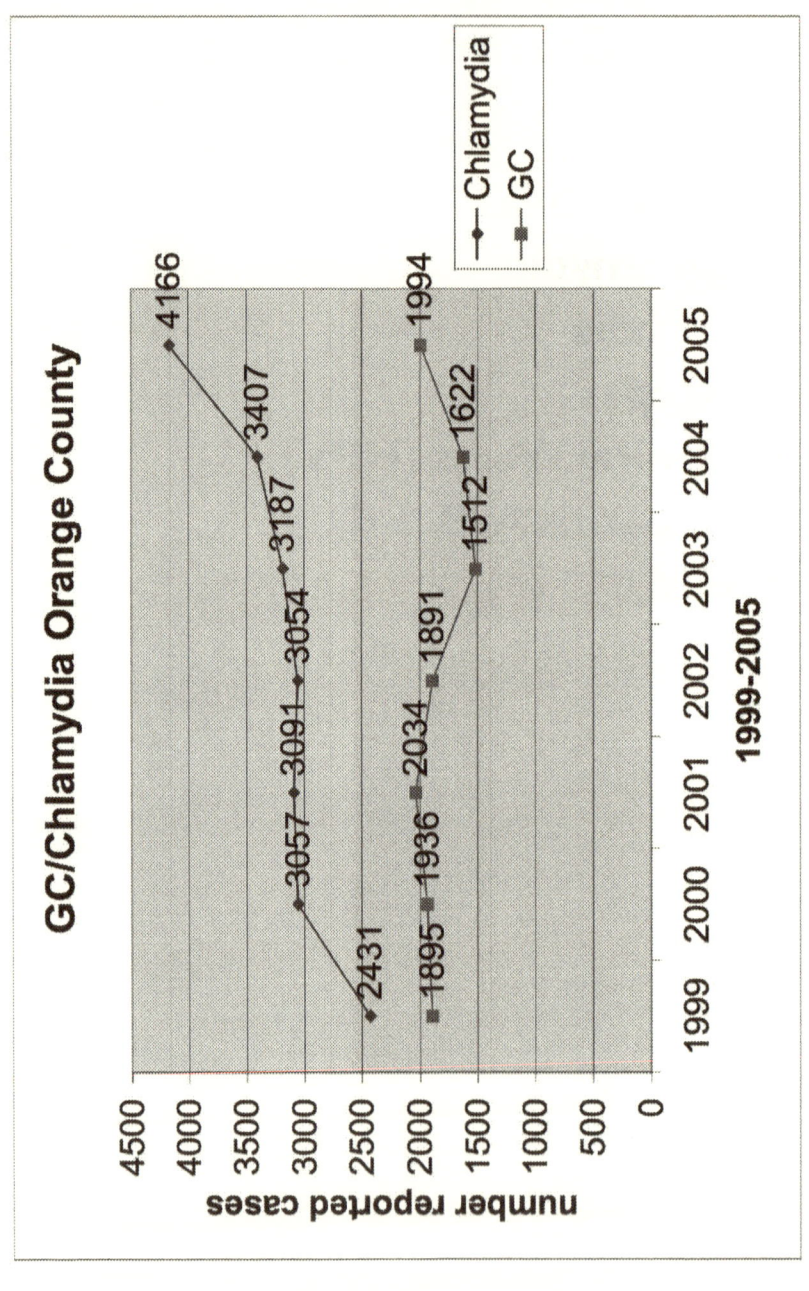

GC/Chlamydia Orange County

number reported cases

1999-2005

Chlamydia: 2431, 3057, 3091, 3054, 3187, 3407, 4166
GC: 1895, 1936, 2034, 1891, 1512, 1622, 1994

Years: 1999, 2000, 2001, 2002, 2003, 2004, 2005

Legend: Chlamydia, GC

Gonorrhea

- **From Greek "gonos" (seed) + "rhoea" (to flow)**
- **Term "clap" derived from French "clapiers" (rabbit warrens - houses of prostitution used during Middle Ages)**
- **Organism: *Neisseria gonorrhoeae***

Clinical Manifestations

- **Urethritis - MALE**

  - **Incubation: 1-14 days (usually 2 - 5 days)**
  - **Sx: Dysuria and urethral discharge (5% asymptomatic)**
  - **Complications**

Clinical Manifestations

- **Urogenital infection - FEMALE**

  - **Endocervical canal primary site**
  - **Incubation: unclear; Sx usually in 10 days**
  - **Sx: majority asymptomatic; may have vaginal discharge, dysuria, urination, labial pain/swelling, abdominal pain**
  - **Complications**

Gonorrhea - Pharyngeal Infection

- **Oral sexual contact**
- **Sx: Asymptomatic in > 90%, pharyngitis**

Gonorrhea - Rectal Infections

- **30-50% women w/GC**
- **Approximately 40% infected homosexual males**
- **Sx: usually asymptomatic; may have discharge, pain, constipation**

Gonorrhea - Conjunctivitis

- **Children: ophthalmia neonatorum (1-7d after ROM)**
- **Adults: autoinoculation**

DGI – Skin Lesions

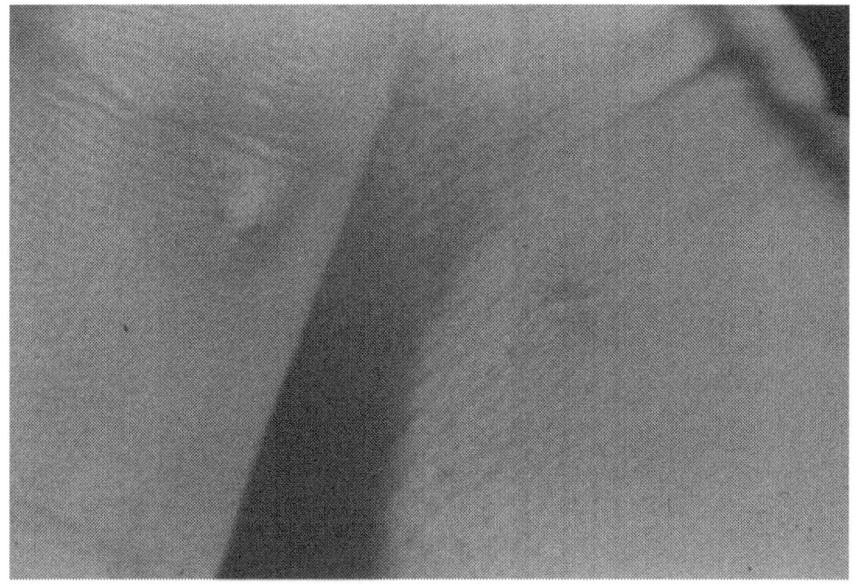

CHLAMYDIA

- is a common sexually transmitted disease (STD) caused by the bacterium, *Chlamydia trachomatis.*

Symptoms

- **Chlamydia, is known as a "silent" disease because about 3/4 of infected women and about 1/2 of infected men have no symptoms.**
- **If symptoms do occur, they usually appear within 1 - 3 weeks after exposure.**

Symptoms

- **Male**
  white discharge from the penis
  burning sensation when urinating

- **Female**
  abnormal vaginal discharge or a
  burning sensation when urinating

ALERT

- **PLEASE turn your head or Shut your eyes ☺ if you are offended by pictures of the male and female sex organs**

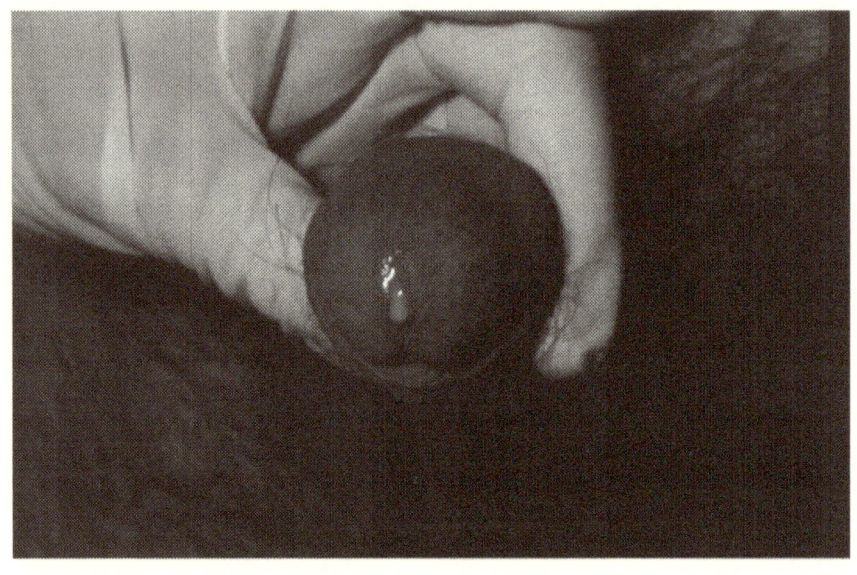

Pelvic Inflammatory Disease

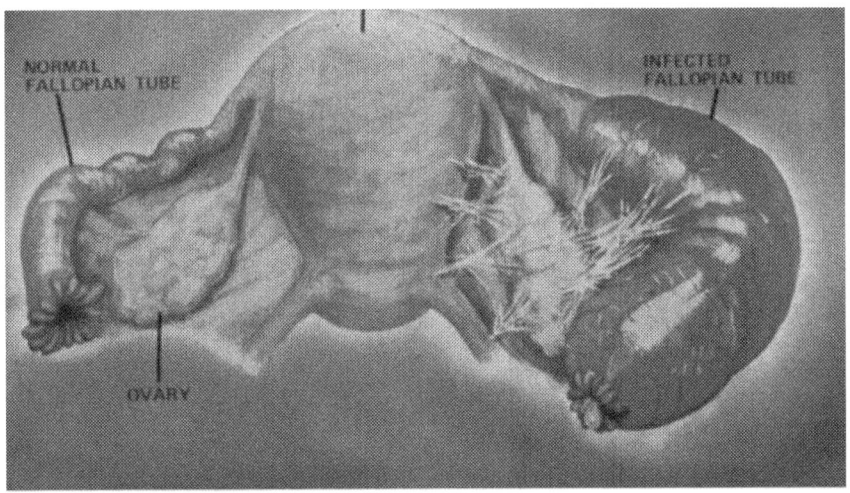

PID - Laparoscopy

Syphilis

- **Syphilis –The Great Imitator**
- **Caused by the organism** *treponema pallidum* **– a spirochete bacteria**
- **Spread sexually by contact with sores or mucous leisions etc.**
- **Incubation 10 – 90 days…**
     Average 3 weeks

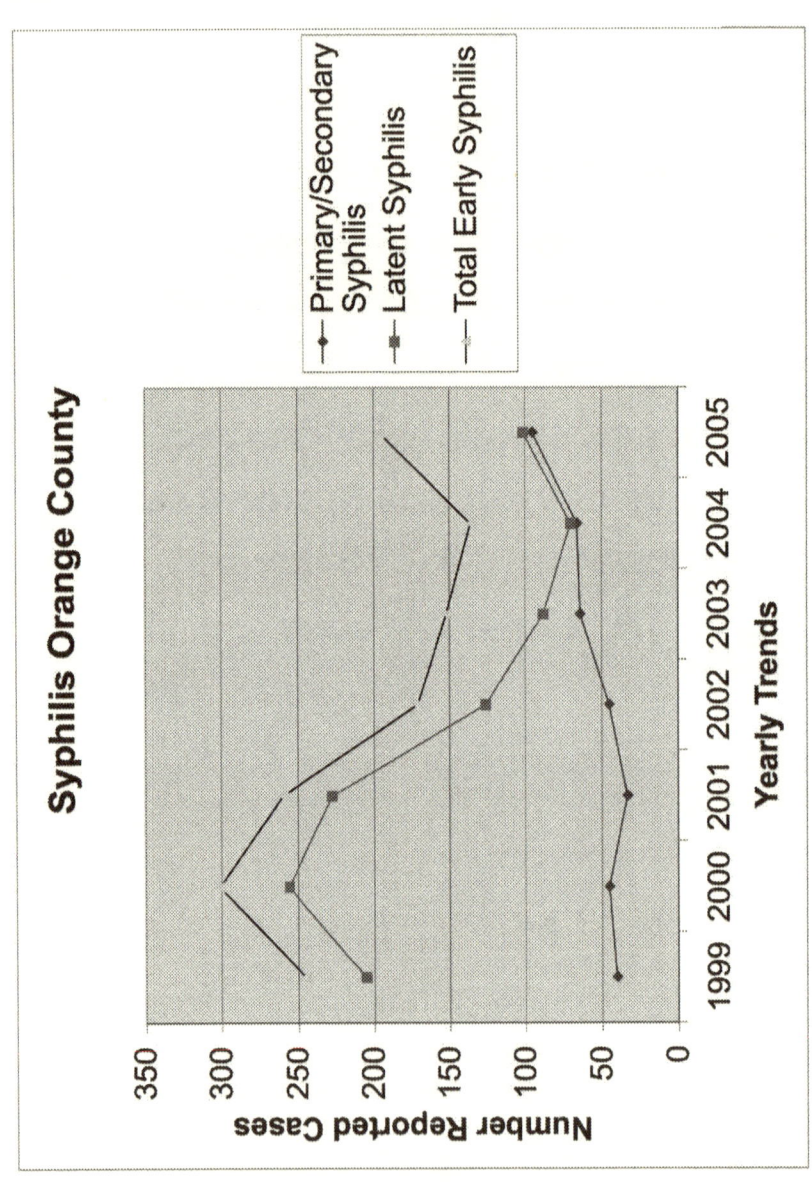

Syphilis Orange County

Legend:
- Primary/Secondary Syphilis
- Latent Syphilis
- Total Early Syphilis

Number Reported Cases (y-axis): 0, 50, 100, 150, 200, 250, 300, 350

Yearly Trends (x-axis): 1999, 2000, 2001, 2002, 2003, 2004, 2005

PRIMARY SYPHILIS

- **Chancre**
  - **early: macule/papule → erodes**
  - **late: clean based, painless, indurated ulcer with smooth firm borders**
  - **unnoticed in 15-30% of patients (anal/vaginal)**
  - **lasts 1-5 weeks, 3 week average**
  - **Appears at site of initial contact**
  - **HIGHLY INFECTIOUS**

ALERT

PLEASE turn your head
or
Shut your eyes ☺

If you feel you might be offended by graphic pictures of genitalia containing examples of syphilis symptoms

Syphilis - Primary

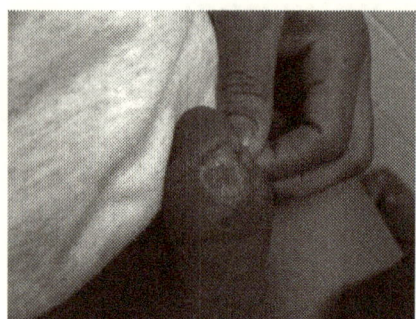

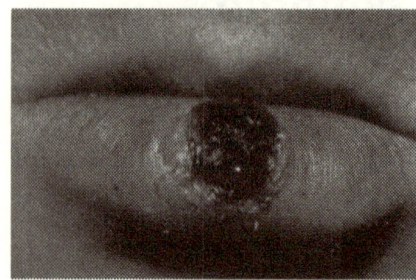

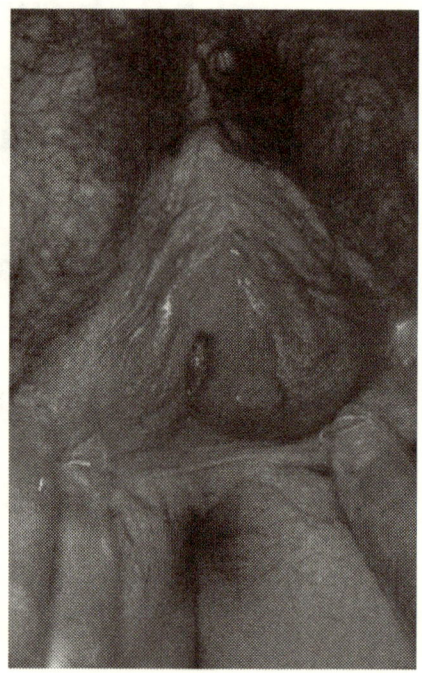

Secondary Syphilis

- spirochetes spread throughout the body
- Usually 2-8 weeks after chancre appears
- Symptoms examples:
  - rash - whole body (includes palms/soles)
  - mucous patches
  - condylomata lata - **HIGHLY INFECTIOUS**
  - Hair loss
- Signs/symptoms 2-6 weeks average 4 weeks
- Symptoms go away even without treatment

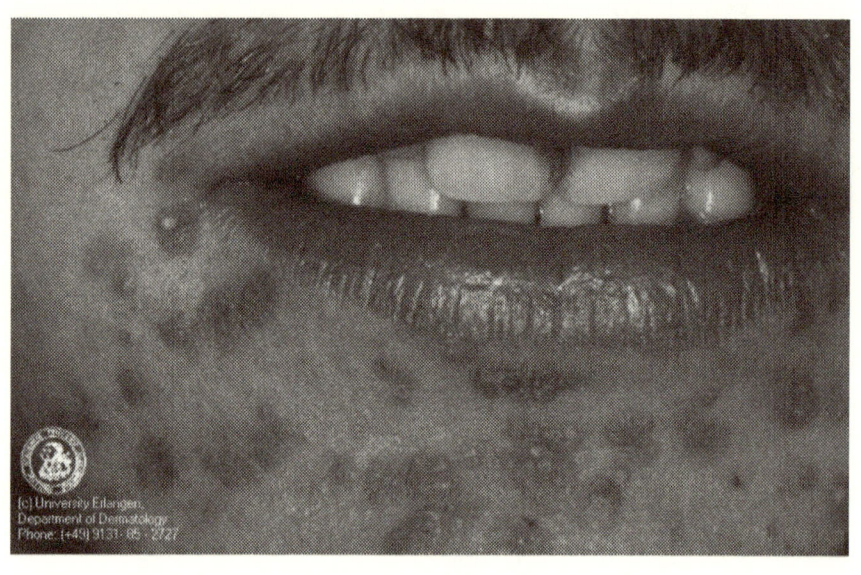

(c) University Erlangen,
Department of Dermatology
Phone: (+49) 9131- 85 - 2727

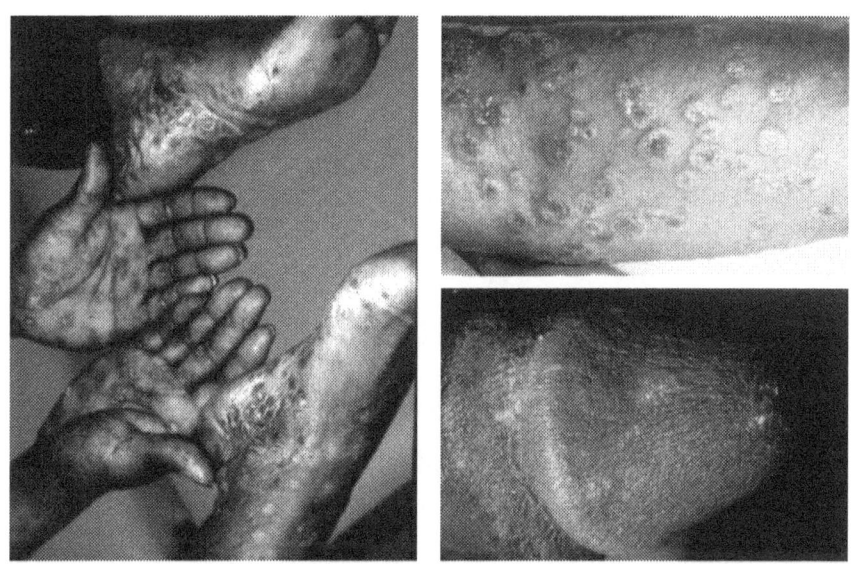

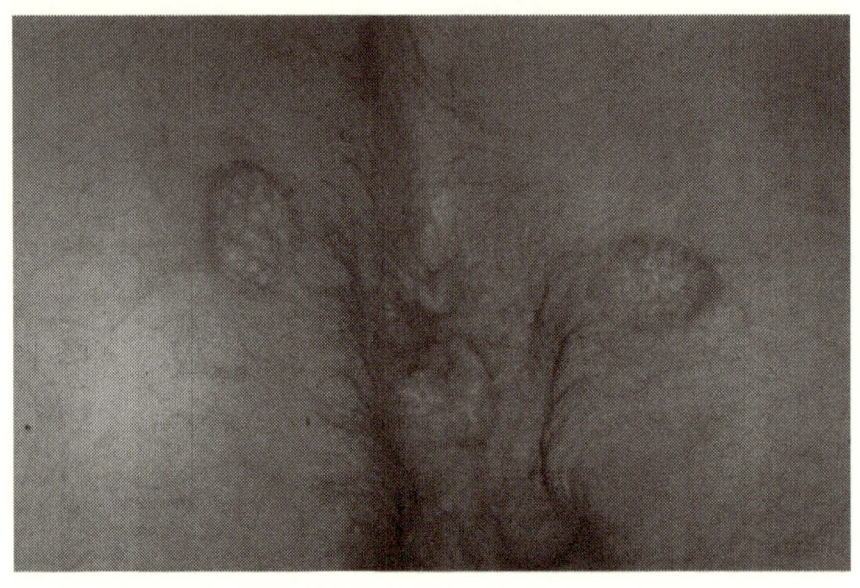

Early Latent Syphilis

- **Infected with Syphilis with no signs or symptoms**
- **Period between primary and secondary syphilis**
- **0-10 weeks –average 4 weeks**
- **After symptoms have disappeared up to one year**
- **NOTE: Late syphilis is untreated syphilis greater than 12 months**

Congenital Syphilis

Hypertropic Skin

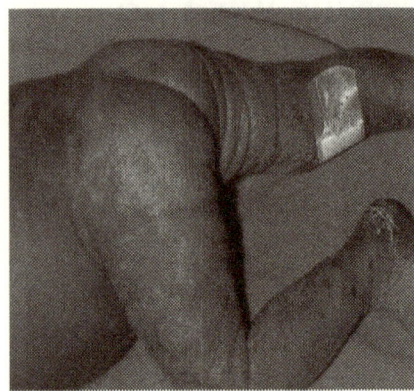

Hemorraoic Snuffles

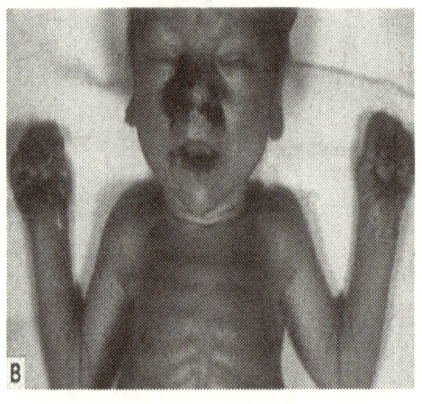

Complications of untreated syphilis

- **Stillbirth in pregnant females**
- **Congenital syphilis (many babies die from major complications)**
- **There are long term complications if adequate treatment not received**
- **Many times, damage done can NOT be corrected even if appropriate medicine is received**
- **Include Blindness, cardiovascular (heart) problems, paresis, insanity, death**

"Syphilis can increase your risk of getting HIV up to 500 times"

Herpes (HSV)

- **20 million people are infected**
- **15% of persons age 15-49 currently infected**
- **6.2 million new infections each year**
- **>50% of sexually active men & women acquire genital HPV infection**

Herpes (HSV)

- Herpes is caused by the herpes simplex viruses type 1 (HSV-1) and type 2 (HSV-2). Most genital herpes is caused by HSV-2.

- Most individuals have no symptoms. When signs do occur, they typically appear as one or more blisters on or around the genitals or rectum which break, leaving tender ulcers (sores) that may take two to four weeks to heal the first time they occur.

- Another outbreak can appear weeks or months after the first, but it almost always is less severe and shorter than the first outbreak.

- Although the infection can stay in the body indefinitely, the number of outbreaks tends to decrease over a period of years.

Best Medicine is
PREVENTION

- **If you see symptoms like those above on you or your partners, see a medical provider immediately.**
- **If infected, inform you partners to seek medical treatment so they will be ok and won't re-infect (give it back to) you**

Human Papillomavirus (HPV) ie: Gential Warts -

- **HPV is the <u>most common</u> STD infection in the US**
- **First infection is usually acquired soon after sexual debut. Infection with multiple types common**
- **Infection is usually transient and not associated with symptoms – 90% of infections clear within 2 years**
- **Persistent HPV infection is cause of cervical cancer as well as other anogenital cancers**
- **100 different types - about 40 types are sexually transmitted**

Genital Warts
Condyloma Acuminata

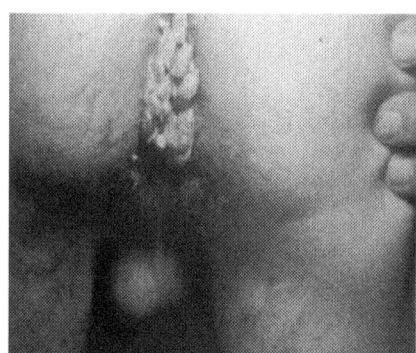 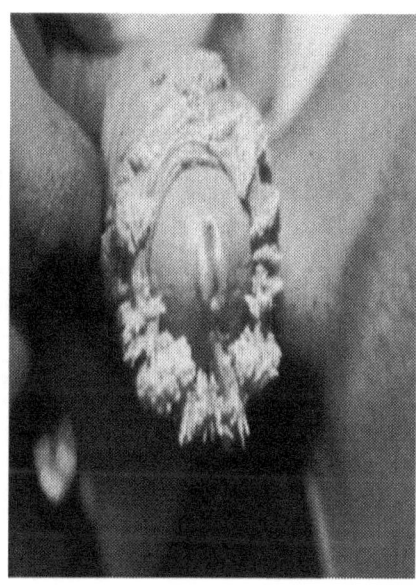

Hepatitis A

- **A liver disease, caused by Hepatitis A virus (HAV), that can affect anyone.**
- **Generally spread by failure to properly wash hands after using the restroom.**
- **Can occur in isolated cases to widespread epidemics**

Hepatitis B

- **Hepatitis B Virus (HBV) attacts the liver.**
- **Can cause lifelong infection, cirrhosis (scarring) of the liver, liver cancer, and death**
- **Easily spread through sexual contact, and exposure to blood or blood products**

Hepatitis C

- **Hepatitis C Virus (HCV) causes liver disease, and is spread primarily by contact with the blood of an infected person.**

HIV/AIDS

- **HIV is primarily spread by:**
- **sexual contact or sharing needles with an infected person**
- **transfusions of infected blood or blood clotting factors.**
- **Babies born to HIV-infected women may become infected before or during birth or through breast-feeding after birth.**

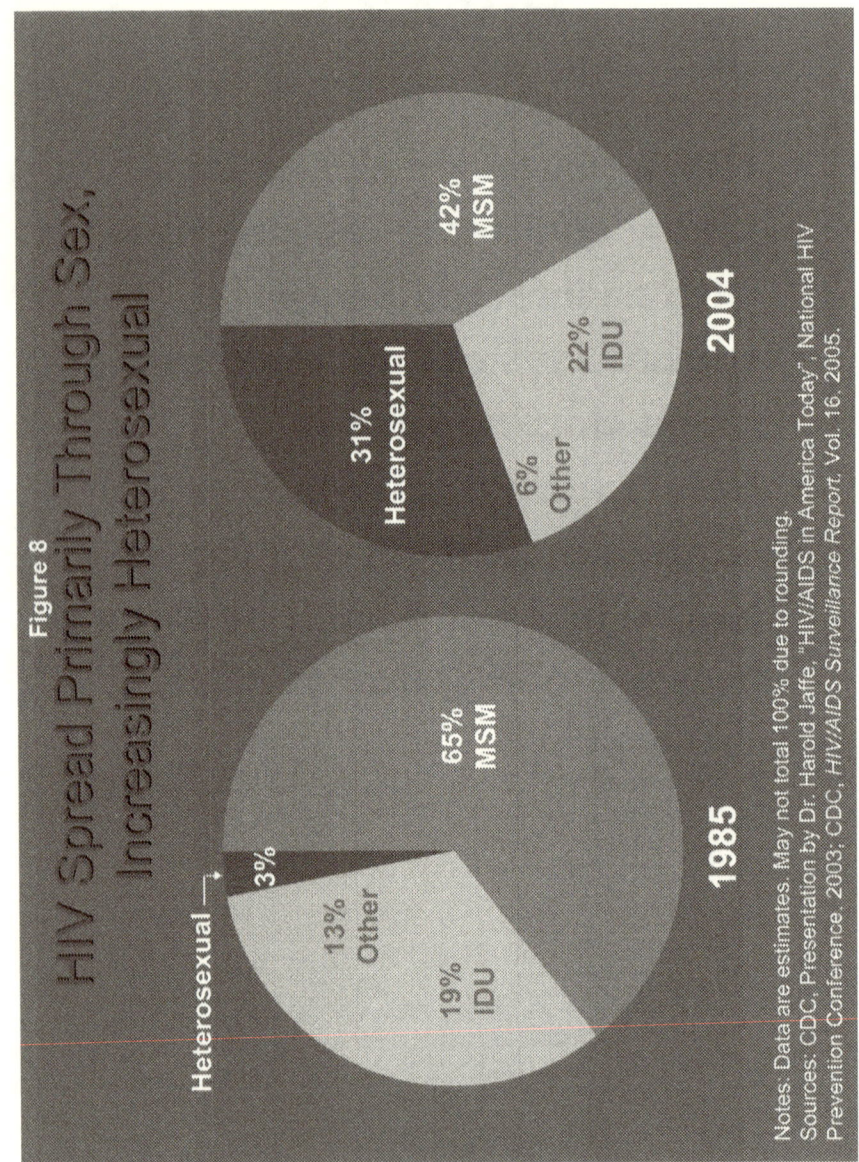

Figure 8

HIV Spread Primarily Through Sex, Increasingly Heterosexual

1985

65% MSM

Heterosexual → 3%

13% Other

19% IDU

2004

42% MSM

31% Heterosexual

6% Other

22% IDU

Notes: Data are estimates. May not total 100% due to rounding.

Sources: CDC, Presentation by Dr. Harold Jaffe, "HIV/AIDS in America Today." National HIV Prevention Conference. 2003; CDC, *HIV/AIDS Surveillance Report*, Vol. 16. 2005.

The U.S. Epidemic: Snapshot of Key Data

New infections each year	**40,000**
People living with HIV/AIDS	**1,039,000 – 1,185,000**
People with HIV/ AIDS not in care	**42 – 59%**
People with HIV who don't know they're infected	**24 – 27%**

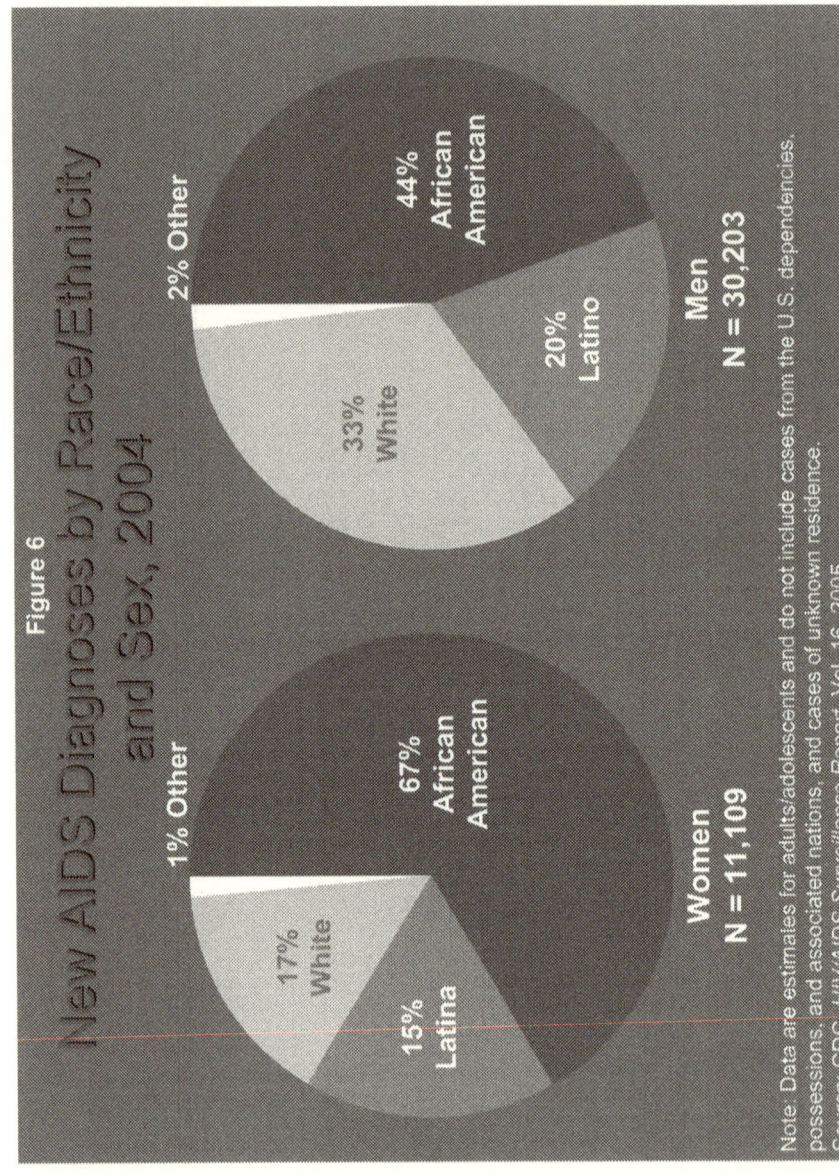

Figure 6

New AIDS Diagnoses by Race/Ethnicity and Sex, 2004

Women
N = 11,109

- 67% African American
- 15% Latina
- 17% White
- 1% Other

Men
N = 30,203

- 44% African American
- 20% Latino
- 33% White
- 2% Other

Note: Data are estimates for adults/adolescents and do not include cases from the U.S. dependencies, possessions, and associated nations, and cases of unknown residence.

Source: CDC. *HIV/AIDS Surveillance Report*, Vol. 16, 2005.

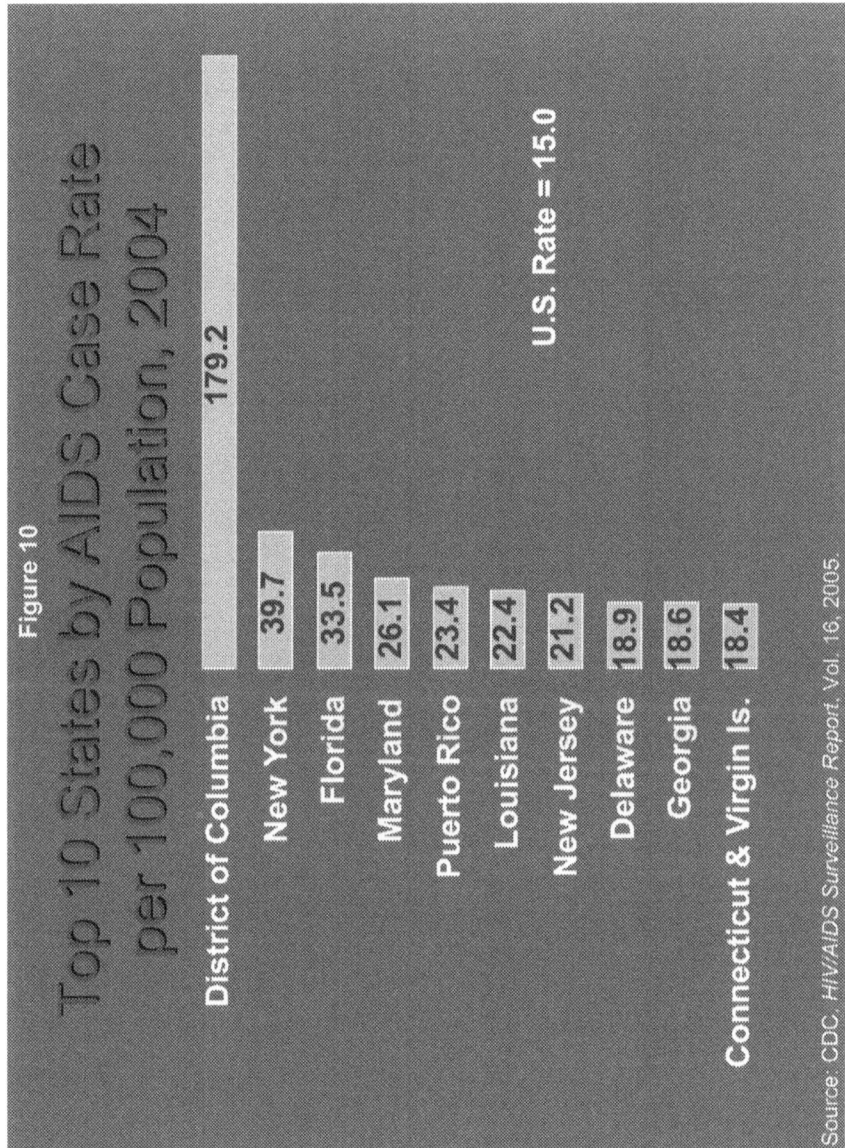

Figure 10

Top 10 States by AIDS Case Rate per 100,000 Population, 2004

District of Columbia	179.2
New York	39.7
Florida	33.5
Maryland	26.1
Puerto Rico	23.4
Louisiana	22.4
New Jersey	21.2
Delaware	18.9
Georgia	18.6
Connecticut & Virgin Is.	18.4

U.S. Rate = 15.0

Source: CDC. *HIV/AIDS Surveillance Report,* Vol. 16, 2005.

CDC's "Advancing HIV Prevention: New Strategies for A Changing Epidemic", 2003

- Aims to:
  - reduce barriers to early diagnosis of HIV
  - increase access to quality medical care, treatment, and ongoing prevention services for with HIV.
- Four Main Strategies
  - Incorporate HIV testing as a routine part of care in traditional medical settings
  - Implement new models for diagnosing HIV infections outside medical settings (e.g., rapid testing)
  - Prevent new infections by working with people diagnosed with HIV and their partners
  - Further decrease mother-to-child HIV transmission

Key Summary Points about the Domestic Epidemic

- **25 years of HIV/AIDS**
- **Tremendous successes in the U.S. including**
  - **significant reduction in new infections since the 1980s**
  - **antiretroviral treatment and people living longer**
  - **reduction in mother to child transmission**
- **But the U.S. epidemic is not over - troubling signs, potential increases among some populations**
- **Impact varies across country – complex & "local"**
  - **Minority Americans, particularly African Americans, women, young people, men who have sex with men**
- **Many challenges remain for prevention, care, treatment, and research**

STD Prevention

- **Abstain from sex**
- **Monogamous Relationship**
- **Get tested on a regular basis (2x year)**
- **Use condoms (male & female condoms are available)**
- **Dental Dams (Saran wrap)**
- **Finger cots**

CHAPTER 5

ACHIEVING YOUR GOALS
WHAT IS A GOAL?

In understanding how to achieve our goals, we must know what a goal is.

A goal, is the object toward which effort is directed. A goal, is different for everybody. It could be as small as adding cranberries to your diet, or as big as planning to be a millionaire.

A goal, is thriving to reach and succeed in an area of our lives that is "broken" or "needs improvement".

We all need improvement, wouldn't you say? Everything significant, begins with a vision and a first step.

HOW DO WE SET GOALS?

Before we start I would like you to ask yourself:
- Am I the person I want to be?
- Where do I want to invest my energies?
- What is holding me back?

Lists of example are below to set you on your way.

1. LIFE IMPROVEMENTS.
   - Goal setting starts as realistic goals of positive life improvements such as:
   - Incorporating 2x a week walking and exercise 15 minutes a day, striving to increase to 3x a week, 30 minutes a day.

2. CHANGE OUR MIND AND ATTITUDE.
   - Our mind can be our worst enemy or a good friend.
   - Our thoughts can either build self-esteem, or undermine our sense of self worth.
   - If we continue to corrupt our thinking or indulge in negative confessions about ourselves, we will inevitably destroy our self-esteem.
   - We must discipline our thoughts.
   - Decide to act.
   - We must accept our life situation.
   - We must always think positive.
   - Positive thoughts attract.
   - Negative thoughts repel.
   - Prepare yourself to face anything.
   - Plant your picture in your mind.
   - Control the nature of your pictures.
   - Positive thinking, can dispel fear and worry.
   - Listen, to the voice within.

Every action, every thought, starts off in the mind.
   - Lack of sleep,affects it.
   - Ill health, affects it.
   - Bad Company, affects it.
   - Negativity, affects it.
   - Fantasying, affects

We have the power to open or shut that door. No one else can.

Make progress slowly, but surely.

NEVER, use your positive approach for selfish purposes.

There is a solution to every problem. Scripture, reminds us to set our mind on those things, which are positive, true, honest, just, pure, lovely and good. We must guard our thought life. This positive power, can be proved by the teaching of the Bible. Read and determine for yourself whether or not the proofs I offer, stand by themselves. Share, your good fortune with others.

Your mind can heal you, if you believe it, it is so!

The message I share with you today is in every book, look for it!

Become face to face with yourself.

Can we do it?

Absolutely!

Scripture indicates:

"I can do all things through Christ who strengthens me"
(Phil 4:13.)

It's ok to lose a few battles, but we don't have to lose the war. All of us are here today to win the war. So Congratulations to all!!

3. CHANGE OUR HABITS
   - A habit is a practice or behavior. It is a repetitive behavior. A habit implies something we have learned to do unconsciously and often compulsively; something done repeatedly.
   - Do you know a habit can be harmless or life threatening? It is considered a character weakness.
   - Habits can be extremely important.
   - Habits have a tremendous impact upon the course of our lives and our destiny.

Let me illustrate some examples below of the chain of events:

- We give birth to a thought, which becomes a deed.
- The birth to a deed, becomes a habit.
- The birth of the habit, becomes our destiny.

Think about it.

So from these few examples, we have established that the many decisions and choices in our lives, lye in our hands. No one is responsible for our lives but us.

4. BETTER HEALTH CHOICES

Please note: I am not a physician. I am an individual, simply providing useful information and suggestions to take into consideration. Always consult with your physician on the appropriate vitamins and supplements.

- Abstinence is the only way to protect yourself 100%. However, being realistic and being aware that sex outside marriage does exist, I can only recommend that practicing safe sex is crucial in halting this disease.
- Simple life changes, can keep us healthy so we can enjoy everyday of our lives.
- Take our prescription medication as prescribed.
- Keep our immunizations current.
- Attend support groups, to learn and share information.
- Keep blood pressure to 115/76
- Walk 15 to 30 minutes a day. Also try to incorporate some lunges, crunches and push-ups.
- Park our cars further from the shopping centers.
- Eat more fish. Fish, is found to decrease inflammation.
- Get a good night sleep. Women, are required 6 to 7 hours and men 8 hours.

- Always stimulate the mind. Reading, watching educational programs, Seminars, are all good ways to stimulate the mind. Make every moment count.
- Manage finances. Live within your means. Living over our limit, will cause extreme stress.
- Learn stress reduction techniques. Lie on the floor and breathe.
- Pay attention to the breaths and the diaphragm rise up and fall.

My favorite technique is "Crunching you face". Try it. Crunch your face, and see if you are able to think about anything. You can't. When I perform this technique, my mind goes blank. It really helps me forget my stress.

- Read food labels.
- Wash hands often.
- Wash vegetables, and fruit in lukewarm water before eating.
- Have 9 servings, (1 serving is a fist size) of fruits, and vegetables daily.
- Beware of the word "Enriched".
- Beware of the word "Corn Syrup"
- Take the right amount of vitamin D (recommended-400 iu). Vitamin D, can be found in Milk, Orange Juice, and also a half hour of sunlight.
- Folic Acid, (400mg) in required for women. Men, are required 300mg. Pregnant women require 800mg or more. It has been found, that women who take Folic Acid supplements before they become pregnant, reduce the risk of birth defects.
- Omega 3: found in olive oil and avocados.
- Call a friend.

- Flossing, and brushing daily, keeps bacteria from forming in the intestines.
- Change toothbrush- every month and after a cold.
- Calcium Magnesium- is found to help with bones and joints.
- Vitamin A, (2500mg or less): Note: too much Vitamin A can cause liver and kidney problems.
- 1 ounce of nuts daily-preferably walnuts.
- Enjoy healthy fat before meals. Have an avocado spread with whole grain.
- Find beauty in the world, and in your life.

Don't we want to be in control of our actions? I know I do.

Decide today to set up goals.

If you are a visual person like myself, you can use the example listed below.

- Draw a large circle on a piece of paper.
- Write on the top of the paper "2006 Goals".
- Draw a line down the middle of the circle.
- Draw a line across the circle (Left to right).
- Draw a line diagonally in the circle.
- Draw another diagonal line in the opposite direction.

You should have a circle that looks like a pizza pie or a pie chart.

In each space on your pie chart, write a goal you would like to accomplish, (fill all the spaces on your chart).

Congratulations, you have just empowered yourself and had set up your goals!

Place this goal sheet, in a place you will be able to view daily.

When completing a goal, highlight the space on your goal chart.

When you complete your goal chart, you will realize how much one person can achieve.

Final note:
Don't get discouraged, if you were unable to reach your goals that day, that month or that year. The great thing is, you can always start with a new day everyday!

CHAPTER 6

LEARN TO TEACH OTHERS

In order for you to teach others, you need to lean and categorize your gifts.

We all have "Gifts of Service".

The Gifts of Service has certain characteristics such as:

- A strong desire to be with other people.
- Disregards any weariness on their part.
- Views practical needs.
- Loves others to achieve.
- Has difficulty saying no.
- Meets needs quickly.
- Loves short range projects.
- Needs approval and recognition.
- Alerts to likes and dislikes
- Operates best using their gifts.
- Tendency to feel inadequate.
- Shows commitment.
- Gets things done.
- Hospitable.
- Generous.
- Joyful.
- Flexible.
- Available.
- Possesses endurance.

This list is just to name some examples of individual personal traits, and characteristics.

Without a doubt, each individual will have one or more of these gifts.

If you don't wouldn't you like to?

Once you have identified your personal character or gifts, you need to practice and develop it. Developing your gifts, is not difficult. It takes time, patience, and love for yourself, and others. You must invest time in getting to know yourself better.

Surround yourself, in environments, and places where you can exercise your gifts.

Once you have mastered your gifts, go and spread it to others. Share it, and teach others through word of mouth, friends, family, Churches, gatherings, events, newspapers, web pages. The methods of transmitting your gifts, are endless.

I would like to challenge you today, to spend time with yourself. Find out who you really

are. Use the many wonderful resources, and web links available at the end of the book to help you.

Seek the many gifts each one of us obtains.

Remember:

"Your life counts".

Share your gifts with the world!

"You will know them by their fruit" (Mat 7:20)

CHAPTER 7

POINTS OF REFERENCE & DISCLAIMER

POINTS OF REFERENCE:

(-1)   Holy Bible-King James Version/Study Helps Concordance/ Seminars Unlimited Edition

(-2)   CDC- Center for Disease Control and Prevention
http://www.cdc.gov/hiv/pubs/faq/faq1.htm

(-3)   HIV/AIDS Timeline
http://www.co.monterey.ca.us/health/CommunityHealth/ pdfs/123101HIVTimeline.pdf

(-4)   MMWR Weekly July 09, 1982/31 (26);353-4,360-1
http://www.cdc.gov/mmwr/preview/mmwrhtml/00001123. htm

(-5)   CDC (1982) ' Kaposi's Sarcoma (KS), Pneumocystis Carinii Pneumonia (PCP), and Other Opportunistic Infections (01): Cases Reported to CDC as of July 8'

(-6)   Frontline: the age of aids: interview: Franklin Graham/PBS
http://www.pbs.org/wgbh/pages/frontline/aids/interviews/ graham.html

(-7)   MMWR Weekly (1982) 'Opportunistic infections and Kaposi's Sarcoma among Haitians in the United States', July 9,31 (26); 353-4,360-1 MMWR Weekly (1982) 'Epidemiologic notes and Reports Pneumocystis carinii Pneumonia among persons with hemophilia A', July 16, 31(27); 365-7,).

(-8)   NewScientist.com-Timeline: HIV/AIDS- 01 July- New Scientist
http://www.newscientist.com/popuparticle.ns?id=in79

Sources: New Scientist, WHO, UNAIDS, New York Times, The Henry J. Kaiser Family Foundation, AIDS Action, AVERT.

(-9) NOW. Science & Health. Global Health: America's Response. Aids Policy Timeline/PBS.　Sources: The Kaiser Family Foundation, UNAIDS, THE ECONOMIST; WHO. http://www.pbs.org/now/science/aidstimeline.html.

(-10) National Institue of Health-timeline 1981-1988- http://www.history.nih.gov/NIHInOwnWords/docs/page_26.html

(-11) Avert-The history of AIDS- http://www.avert.org/his87_92.htm Purvis A. (1990) 'Rumania's other tragedy', The Time Magazine, February 19 http://www.avert.org/his87_92.htm

(-12) FDA- HIV AIDS Historical Time Line 1981-1990 http://www.fda.gov/oashi/aids/miles81.html

(-13) U. S. Food and Drug Administration FDA Brochure: 1992 http://www.cfsan.fda.gov/~dms/aidseat.html

(-14) United States Department of Agriculture Food Safety and Inspection Service http://www.fsis.usda.gov/Fact_Sheets/Food_Safety_for_Persons_with_AIDS/index.asp

(-15) Avert-The history of AIDS- http://www.avert.org/his87_92.htm Marklink R.G (1998) 'Remembrance of Jonathan Mann' in www.iapac.org accessed 22/5/02

(-16) Avert- The history of AIDS- http://www.avert.org/his87_92.htm Sawyer E. (1998) 'Tribute: Mann of the hour' in www.poz.com accessed 22/5/02

(-17) qAIDSinfo-a Service of the U.S. Department of Health and Human Services http://www.aidsinfo.nih.gov/ContentFiles/ApprovedMedstoTreatHIV_FS_en.pdf http://www.fda.gov/oashi/aids/virals.html

(-18) MMWR Weekly-June 2, 2006/55(21);585-589 CDC. Evolution of HIV prevention programs---United States, 1981--2006. MMWR 2006;55:597--602.

144

http://www.cdc.gov/mmwr/preview/mmwrhtml/
mm5521a1.htm?s_cid=mm5521a1_e

(-19) MMWR Weekly June 2, 2006/55(21);585-589 Twenty-Five Years of HIV/AIDS---United States, 1981-2006 http://www.cdc.gov/mmwr/preview/mmwrhtml/mm5521a1.htm?s_cid=mm5521a1_e   Presidential Advisory Council on HIV/AIDS. Achieving an HIV-free generation: recommendations for a new American HIV strategy. Washington, DC: US Department of Health and Human Services; 2006.

Disclaimer:

VENUS PEREZ is the copyright owner of this book.

The Author of this book and the accompanying materials used her best efforts in preparing this book. Every effort has been made to accurately represent our book and it's potential.

VENUS PEREZ hopes that the information in this book will be valuable and useful to readers. Nothing in this book constitutes advice. The information is not intended to be a substitute for professional advice. Your use of the information contained in these pages, however, is at your sole risk. All information on these pages is provided "as –is", without any warranty.

The information contained in this book is strictly for educational purposes. Therefore, if you wish to apply ideas contained in this book, you are taking full responsibility for your actions.

The testimony and examples used are exceptional results, don't apply to the average reader and are not intended to represent or guarantee that anyone will achieve the same or similar results.

Each reader's success depends on his or her background, dedication, desire and motivation.

VENUS PEREZ will not be liable for any damages you may sustain by using this information, whether direct, indirect, special, incidental or consequential, even if it has been advised of the possibility of such damages.

The author does not warrant the effectiveness or applicability of any sites listed or linked to this book.

All sites and links are for information purposes only and are not warranted for content, accuracy or any other implied or explicit purpose.

VENUS PEREZ makes no express or implied representations, warranties, or guarantees with regard to the appropriateness, accuracy, sufficiency, correctness, veracity, value, completeness, or timeliness or such information.

VENUS PEREZ expressly disclaims all warranties of any kind, whether express or implied, including, but not limited to the implied warranties of fitness for a particular purpose and non-infringement.

Any pages in this book printed for educational purposes its shall be the responsibility of the person so doing to comply with the laws to the state or nation within which the material shall be used.

The terms of this disclaimer will be governed by and construed in accordance with United States law and both VENUS PEREZ and the individual users submit to the non-exclusive jurisdiction of the United States courts.

This book is © copyright by VENUS PEREZ. No part of this may be copied, or changed in any format, sold, or used in any way other than what is outlined with this book under any circumstances.

www.ingramcontent.com/pod-product-compliance
Lightning Source LLC
Chambersburg PA
CBHW031324290526
45784CB00014B/996